How to Run a Personal Record

How to Run a Personal Record

Cover the Ground in Front of You Faster Than Ever Before

Dave Kuehls

A PERIGEE BOOK

A PERIGEE BOOK
Published by the Penguin Group
Penguin Group (USA) Inc.
375 Hudson Street, New York, New York 10014, USA
Penguin Group (Canada), 90 Eglinton Avenue East, Suite 700, Toronto, Ontario M4P 2Y3, Canada
(a division of Pearson Penguin Canada Inc.) • Penguin Books Ltd., 80 Strand, London WC2R 0RL,
England • Penguin Group Ireland, 25 St. Stephen's Green, Dublin 2, Ireland (a division of Penguin
Books Ltd.) • Penguin Group (Australia), 250 Camberwell Road, Camberwell, Victoria 3124,
Australia (a division of Pearson Australia Group Pty. Ltd.) • Penguin Books India Pvt. Ltd.,
11 Community Centre, Panchsheel Park, New Delhi—110 017, India • Penguin Group (NZ),
67 Apollo Drive, Rosedale, North Shore 0632, New Zealand (a division of Pearson New Zealand Ltd.) •
Penguin Books (South Africa) (Pty.) Ltd., 24 Sturdee Avenue, Rosebank, Johannesburg 2196, South Africa

Penguin Books Ltd., Registered Offices: 80 Strand, London WC2R 0RL, England

While the author has made every effort to provide accurate telephone numbers and Internet addresses at
the time of publication, neither the publisher nor the author assumes any responsibility for errors, or for
changes that occur after publication. Further, the publisher does not have any control over and does not
assume any responsibility for author or third-party websites or their content.

First edition: January 2009

Library of Congress Cataloging-in-Publication Data

Kuehls, Dave.
   How to run a personal record : cover the ground in front of you faster than ever before / Dave Kuehls.— 1st ed.
      p.   cm.
   Includes index.
   ISBN 978-0-399-53478-2
   1. Running—Training.   I. Title.
   GV1061.5.K844 2009
   796.42'4—dc22   2008031122

PRINTED IN THE UNITED STATES OF AMERICA

10   9   8   7   6   5   4   3   2   1

PUBLISHER'S NOTE: Outdoor recreational activities are by their very nature potentially hazardous. All
participants in such activities must assume the responsibility for their own actions and safety. If you have
any health problems or medical conditions, consult with your physician before undertaking any outdoor
activities. The information contained in this guidebook cannot replace sound judgment and good decision
making, which can help reduce risk exposure, nor does the scope of this book allow for disclosure of all the
potential hazards and risks involved in such activities. Learn as much as possible about the outdoor recreational activities in which you participate, prepare for the unexpected, and be cautious. The reward will be
a safer and more enjoyable experience.

Most Perigee books are available at special quantity discounts for bulk purchases for sales promotions,
premiums, fund-raising, or educational use. Special books, or book excerpts, can also be created to fit
specific needs. For details, write: Special Markets, Penguin Group (USA) Inc., 375 Hudson Street, New York,
New York 10014.

Contents

Introduction

Young and old. Fast and slow. 5K and 10K runners and marathoners. Olympic runners and recreational runners. They are all out there, pursuing it, relentlessly, every weekend in road races and marathons. It's not a victory—though a very select few will be gunning for that. And it's not a finisher's medal—though some will have that in mind. What most runners are thinking about when they stand at the starting line, whether they recognize the terminology or not, is this: "I want to run a PR."

What's a PR? That's a good question. It's an abbreviation that's been working its way through the running community. It stands for "personal record." Originally, PR was a term used in track and field when a runner—in the 100 meters to the 10,000 meters—ran a time faster than he or she had before, and so on the results sheet the letters P and R (PR) would appear in the column next to the finishing time to indicate such an effort. Olympic athletes ran a lot of PRs in their careers, and many got financially rewarded for those efforts each and every time they occurred. Today, a variety of runners use it to describe how they want to cover the distance in front of them faster than they ever have before, to set a personal record.

Take, for example, Mary. She has run six 5Ks in her running career (she just started running two years ago), and her best time for the distance is 27 minutes and 45 seconds. Mary is hoping to better that time in a local 5K this weekend—to set a personal record, or as many runners refer to it, to PR.

Then there is Dan. He took up running four years ago and has completed three marathons, with a best time of 4 hours, 28 minutes, and 17 seconds. Dan is training for the New York City Marathon and hoping to break that time with a more ambitious goal—to run under 4 hours, to PR.

But wanting a PR and knowing how to set a new one, do not necessarily go hand in hand. Mary, for instance, just added one run to her weekly schedule, in hopes that it would take her to a PR. It didn't. And Dan hit the track early and often in his marathon training schedule. The result? A pulled hamstring and Achilles tendonitis that stopped his marathon training cold.

The plain truth of the matter is that most runners who are fairly new to the sport and ambitious about running faster times, as well as many veteran runners who have been flirting with faster times for years, have little clue about how to set a realistic PR. Their approaches will be haphazard. In training, they will try one thing one week (maybe all-out sprints to get faster) and another thing the next week (a run that's really long for them). And then, on the third week, they may expect to race at a level they have never been at before. During the race things get no better. They will inevitably sprint out at the gun and fall into a fast pace, a pace they can only keep up for a short while. Or they will start much slower than they are capable of, holding that pace until the finish line is in sight, and then sprint in for all they are worth. In short, they are doomed to failure—and worse, an inevitable deep frustration with the sport that can cause them to quit running and take up bowling instead.

That's where this book comes in.

If you want to PR, this book will help you focus your training and racing so you can run your goal time for whatever race distance you select. You'll find a solid, time-tested, three-pronged training approach that's sure to get the most out of your ability, laying out specific training programs for the four most popular PR time goals (for example, 45, 50, 55, and 60 minutes for the 10K) in the four most popular racing distances (the 5K, 10K, half marathon, and marathon). It also includes race-day strategies designed to shave precious minutes and seconds from the finish-line clock, and discussions of all the important topics (diet, gear, stretches, etc.) and how they relate to your PR quest.

In short, this book will become your personal trainer in your quest to run a PR.

Not-So-Smart Things People Have Tried to Improve Their Times

Running with ankle weights

Running with hand weights

Running relentless wind sprints

Running backward

Running with a dog

Crash dieting

Running with a parachute

Racing on a downhill course

Cutting the course

Starting their watches at the 1-mile mark

CHAPTER 1

Are You Ready to Run a Personal Record?

Is this you?

You took up running three years ago, and in that time you have run half a dozen races. At first you raced them simply to participate and to finish, but now you are up for a new challenge. The local 10K is coming around again, and you want to see if you can run a time that is faster than you have ever run before.

You want to PR.

When you are ready to include PR in your running lexicon, it means one thing: You are ready for the pursuit. Let me back up a little. In racing there are a lot of carrots to go after: overall trophies, age-group plaques or mugs, relay-member ribbons. Longtime runners will crowd their mantels or stuff their basements with all these awards. Yet if you were to pull them aside and ask them which of their running achievements meant the most to them, they would invariably answer with the running achievements that come with no commemorative piece of hardware, only an internal pat on the back: their PRs.

Why is this? Why does the PR have a hold on runners like no other goal or achievement?

PRs resonate because 99 percent of us take up running to compete with one person above all others—no, not Jill or Joe. That person is our self.

Think about it. Each run you took when you were starting out—a 2 miler, a 3 miler—was a competition with yourself. (*Can I do this?*) And even today, every time you go for a run, it is still, in essence, a minicompetition with yourself. That's because each time you stride out, rather than slow down and walk, you are defeating that voice inside your head that says one thing over and over: "Quit."

The PR, then, means taking this competition with our selves to its extreme—it's what we do when we can take each stride without stopping and complete the distance set before us: We want to see how fast we can go.

The hunt for PRs can keep your racing fresh and vital for years. Each January, as you lay out your running year, you will have a goal time to shoot for in all your racing categories. And at the starting line of any race—be it a local 10K with sixty runners or a big-city marathon with ten thousand—you will have a goal that's unique to you, that's dependent only on your two legs and lungs.

So, are you ready to run a PR?

The Commitment

The term "PR" does not cross the Atlantic. The British don't use the letters *PR* to indicate a personal record. In fact, they have a completely different phrase and abbreviation: personal best and PB.

There is a difference. "Personal best" has always seemed to me to be a step or two removed from "personal record." Think about it: personal record or personal best? To do your "personal best" is not the same thing as setting a "personal record." (The derivation of "personal best" might have something to do with the amateur roots of the sport in Britain, and the perception that the sport shouldn't be taken too seriously.)

What does this mean to you?

It means that when you are ready to step forward and make the commitment to going after a PR, you are really committing to something. You are not simply standing on the starting line trying to achieve your "personal best," not simply trying at that moment in time. Instead, you are after something that will be monumental enough to put down in a records book, to take with you into posterity. Achieving a personal record is not something that will be accomplished by happenstance. It means stepping forward on day one with a specific goal in mind and working toward that end: your PR.

This will take time and effort. The PR schedules in this book are all four months in length. That's four months when you are training to PR in a marathon or half marathon, a 10K or a 5K. You'll need four months so you can go through the three training phases that are the cornerstone for any PR attempt. That attempt will not be easy. (What is the point in devoting four months of training to something you can do by simply going through the motions?) But I'll help you pick a PR goal that is both challenging and within your reach.

Levels of Running Pursuit

Runner's goals change over time. What follows is a typical progression for a runner over the years.

Beginner
Training: getting your feet wet
Racing goals: to finish

Transitional
Training: start to experiment on your own, a bit haphazard
Racing goals: want to run faster, yet don't know how

PR
Training: focused
Racing goals: based on current PRs and projected PRs

Your PR pursuit will take a high level of mental, psychological, and physical commitment, one that you have never applied to running before. Sure, you have done workouts and put in the miles, but this time around each workout and mile will be devoted to a specific time goal, a goal that you will only achieve at the end of four months.

Your PR.

The Seven-to-Ten-Year Window

For runners, there is something called the seven-to-ten-year window. What this means is that once you start running you have seven to ten years to keep improving, to get faster. It's not a hard-and-fast rule—we've all heard of runners who have set their personal records fifteen years or more down the line. But most runners have seven to ten years to get across that finish line faster than before. (This time restriction is due in part to natural aging and the slowing down that occurs because of it.)

What does this window mean to your PR quest? That depends. For the purposes of setting your own PR, I suggest reframing the seven-to-ten-year window. Rather than seeing it as the seven to ten years from the first time you first lace up a pair of running shoes and head out the door, think of it as a competitive window—seven to ten years from the time you start being competitive with yourself, when you start chasing PRs.

So, for the most part, that means if you are picking up this book for the first time, you have seven to ten years of the pursuit, no matter what your age. My father picked up running in his early fifties and ran his best times in his late fifties. He kept improving within the window, despite the fact that he was past what most people would consider the prime age for running.

What does this mean for you? It means if you are young runner—or an older runner—you still have plenty of time to set PRs.

CHAPTER 2

How to Pick a PR Goal

Meet Laura. She is twenty-six years old. She picked up running in college to keep the weight off, took a few years off, then started back at it again.

Since that time, she has been running steadily—three or four days a week—for the past two years, and feeling good. Last spring she jumped into a local 5K on the spur of the moment. She crossed the line in 30 minutes and 15 seconds.

This year, however, she wanted to do better—much better. For a goal time she set for herself the task of running 25 minutes. It was an ambitious goal—but, hey, if you are going to go for it, really go for it, right? Laura was convinced that if she just kept plugging away, somehow she would knock 5 minutes off her 5K PR.

She didn't. Race day dawned and by the first mile she was flying, but hurting big time. And by the second mile she had thrown in the towel. Laura crossed the line in 31 minutes and 7 seconds, almost a minute slower than last year's time. Laura went home disappointed, so disappointed that she quit running all together and put back on all the pounds that she lost by diligently running for the past two years.

What Laura did was fail the first test of pursuing a PR: She chose too ambitious of a goal.

Meet Tom. He is thirty-one years old. He started running four years ago—five days a week—and has competed in several road races, from 5Ks to half marathons. Two years ago he finished his first half marathon, in fact. He jogged comfortably most of the way and finished with a time of 2 hours, 15 minutes, and 33 seconds.

The following year he decided to train for another half marathon. During training Tom set for himself a goal time of 2 hours, 15 minutes, and 32 seconds.

That's right. A 1-second PR for a half marathon.

Come race day, Tom found his goal pace and stuck to it. He finished fairly comfortably again and the time on his watch read: 2 hours, 15 minutes, and 32 seconds.

He did it. But all that running for one second?

What is the point of training for a PR—especially one over a half-marathon distance—when the goal you have set is so easily within reach? Remember, Dan jogged his first half marathon in 2 hours, 15 minutes, and 33 seconds.

The goal of this book will be to help you set PRs that have challenged you.

Setting Your PR Time Goal

There are two questions you need to ask yourself when setting your PR time goal: Is it doable? And is it challenging?

By doable, I mean, can you realistically see yourself doing it? Laura's goal of 5 minutes off her 5K best might have seemed like a monumental goal worth achieving, but it was not doable. It was simply wishful thinking.

By challenging, I mean something that will be worth pursuing for several months of training, and something that will be satisfying when you achieve it at the finish line. You want to be inspired through the months of training, and you want to be in a celebratory mood when you finish. Considering his level of fitness, Tom's one-second PR in a half marathon does not fit this bill.

Of course, only you can know for sure if a PR time goal is doable and challenging. To help with that process, analyze your training and talk with other runners who know your ability well. And to further help you decide, the training schedules in this book are set up in time increments according to what is generally accepted as a challenging but doable goal for the recreational runner: 2½-minute improvement for a 5K; 5-minute improvement for a 10K; 10-minute improvement for a half marathon; and a 15-minute improvement for a marathon.

In the next chapter we will go through the three training phases needed when you are preparing to PR—so you can make those improvements.

CHAPTER 3

How to Train for a PR

There is no completely right or wrong way to train—there are training philosophies that work for some, and different training philosophies that work for others. For example, many successful distance runners train at altitude. Many successful distance runners do not train at altitude. There's no one way.

That said, the training philosophy behind this book is based on a solid three-pronged approach that has been used for decades by many runners—elite athletes as well as everyday joggers. The guiding principle is that in order to run fast, to run a PR during a race, you must work through three stages of training: Road Work, Strength Work, and Track Work, which includes a secret workout.

Let's examine the three phases in detail, the three phases that will make up each and every training schedule.

Road Work

Road Work (aka distance work) is often given short shrift—sometimes even overlooked altogether—when a runner is concentrating on running a PR. Training manuals paraphrase the weeks and months of boring distance work a runner needs to do in preparation to race, and this has a tendency to belittle the phase, as though you can get by without it (or at least some of it), causing many runners to try just that. For example, they will be instructed to put in six weeks of Road Work prior to hitting the track, but they cut that down to perhaps three or four and then jump right in.

This is a mistake. Traditionally this phase has been known by other names, like the Endurance Phase, but for this book I have renamed it Road Work for a singular reason: "Road Work" is a boxing term. It refers to the long, slow miles a boxer will put in (often behind a car driven by his trainer), and as any boxer knows, Road Work is vital to his success. It literally gives him the legs to stand on when he is in the ring, particularly in the later rounds. Without Road Work, a boxer cannot compete with another in the ring. And without Road Work, a runner cannot compete with himself during a race.

What Is It?

Road Work consists of the long, slow runs you do exclusively in the first half of your training program. It is also encompasses the runs you do once or twice a week later in your program, during Strength Work and Track Work.

What Does It Do for You?

Road Work builds up a well of endurance that enables you to "race" the distance. It also provides a base upon which you can add strength and speed without breaking down or becoming exhausted.

What Workouts Does It Include?

In this training program, the weekly long run, the midweek medium run, and the short, slow recovery runs in between (which are detailed in the schedules in Chapter 5) make up Road Work.

How Do I Do It?

You should start slow (at a conversational pace, a pace during which you can carry on a conversation) and finish slow. Run on a relatively flat surface (distance, not hills, should be your challenge), and build up the distance of your runs every week or two weeks. This is done by targeting a long run once a week but also by upping the mileage of some of your other runs during the week. The end result is that you gradually cover more miles in your long run and also run more total miles during the week.

What Mental Approach Should I Take to Road Work?

After a few weeks, Road Work can become boring—you are running slow miles every day—and the temptation is to pick it up on some runs and sooner or later you are no longer running long and slow but short and fast, and your eight weeks of Road Work has been cut in half. Therefore, it is helpful to remind yourself of your goal each day during the Road Work phase: to complete the distance at a slow pace. That's because endurance comes from one thing: time spent running.

What Distances for Road Work Should I Expect?

For a long run, expect to work up to 8 miles while training for a 5K, 10 miles while training for a 10K, 16 miles while training for a half marathon, and 23 miles while training for a marathon. For weekly mileage, expect to work up to 30-plus miles a week for a 5K, 35-plus miles a week for a 10K, 40-plus miles a week for a half marathon, and 50-plus for a marathon.

THE ROAD WORK PHASE: THE ESSENTIALS

THE LONG RUN: The long run is the cornerstone workout in the Road Work phase. The long run preferably occurs on Saturday so Sunday can be spent in recovery, and should take place on a flat, soft surface, where your mileage is either well marked along the way or where overall mileage for the route has been measured ahead of time. Routes can include an out-and-back or a loop course. The out-and-back has a definitive halfway mark (and that can be good or bad, depending on how you are running that day) and can be useful on windy days if you can run out into the wind, and back with the wind at your back. This works because as you are tiring in the later miles, you are not running into the wind but with an assist from the wind. Loop courses might be preferable to train on if you are prepping for a half marathon or marathon, because most half marathons and marathons are not out-and-back and you want to simulate the nature of the course. Overall pace is conversational, and the run can be divided into psychological chunks to help you get through it. For example, if a 16-mile long run is thought of in its entirety, it will make the run seem interminable. But if you can mentally divide the distance into two 8-mile chunks or four segments of 4 miles, this will lighten the load.

Also, the longer the long run, the more helpful it will be to run it with a training partner. (See the discussion of training partners in Chapter 4.)

THE MIDWEEK MEDIUM RUN: The midweek medium run is a supplemental run in the Road Work phase. This run generally occurs Wednesday, after you have had adequate time to recover from the last long run and have enough time ahead of you to prepare for the next long run on Saturday. Preferably run on a soft, flat surface, but if you are training for a marathon and race day is coming up, the midweek medium run might be a good time to "hit the road" to simulate the surface conditions of race day. Run at a conversational pace or slightly faster (this is simply the nature of going less distance), yet monitor the run so as not to become too fast. Distances vary depending on your race distance.

THE RECOVERY RUNS: Recovery runs are the short-distance workouts you run on days when you are not engaged in a long run or a medium distance run. Recovery runs should be done on a soft, flat surface (to promote recovery) and run at a conversational pace or slower. There is a big temptation to run recovery runs fast (since they are so short) and this should be avoided at all costs. Without true recovery during your recovery runs, the Road Work phase will break you down in a matter of weeks. In that respect, slow recovery runs are the most important run during Road Work. If you choose to run them too fast, you will not be able to go on.

DAYS OFF: The day, usually Sunday, following the long run is a day off, a day of rest. This is part of the training process, which can be boiled down to this principle: You stress the body during a long run, then you let the body rest and recover so that it grows stronger. The Sunday day off is the first day in a three-day rest cycle, which is as follows: Rest day, recovery run, recovery run. It is also the most crucial. The day following your long run is the day when muscle tissue is at its most sore, tendons are their most tender, and the body is most fatigued. You need to rest. Without it you will be too fatigued to continue training, and eventually break down, becoming injured or ill or both.

STRIDERS: A few weeks into the Road Work phase you will do striders following select recovery runs. Striders are short, 80- to 100-meter runs on a flat, soft surface. They are not sprints, but "pickups" run at a fresh pace. They serve two purposes. They let the legs run faster, after weeks of long, slow running. And they prepare the body for faster work in the Strength Work phase, when you will be running hills and tempo runs.

Strength Work

Strength Work exists as a middleman in the training process. It is transitional in nature—getting the runner from Road Work to Track Work—but vital to the overall training plan.

What Is It?
Strength Work includes hill climbs and tempo runs.

What Does It Do for You?
Strength Work gives you strength—in your legs, arms, and overall cardiovascular system—strength you will need to "keep the pace" during your

race. Strength Work is also a bridge between Road Work and Track Work. By that I mean that Strength Work prepares the body (coming from a lot of long, slow runs) for the exertion of track work. Without Strength Work, the abrupt shift from slow to fast could cause an injury that would end the training program.

What Workouts Does It Include?

Several climbs up a gradual hill and tempo runs of 20 to 40 minutes.

How Do I Do It?

For hills, start at the bottom of the hill and run up it at a brisk, but controlled, pace. For 5Ks and 10Ks you will do four to six repeats. For the half marathon and full marathon you will do six to eight.

For tempo runs, find a flat stretch of trail or road and run steadily at a pace that's "comfortably close" to PR pace for the distance that you are training for. For 5Ks and 10Ks you will run for 20 minutes. For half marathons and marathons you will run for 40 minutes.

What Mental Approach Should I Take to Strength Work?

Strength Work is when you really start to focus on effort in your training. You'll need to prepare yourself before each run for the effort and also keep steady during your runs.

What Distances for Strength Work Should I Expect?

Hill work will amount to a mile or two in total distance; tempo runs of 40 minutes during half marathon and marathon training can cover four to five miles.

THE STRENGTH WORK PHASE: THE ESSENTIALS

HILL WORK: One of the two cornerstone workouts for the Strength Work phase, hills are run on Tuesdays during the week. The key, of course, is finding the right hill. Look for one about 100 to 200 meters long and about the grade of a highway exit ramp, something challenging but not severe. Footing is also important, so some trails may be off limits. Traffic may be another impediment, so some roads may not be ideal. Scout out possible hill work locations while still in your Road Work phase, so as not to be stuck when hill work comes upon you and you are without an adequate hill.

For hill work, after a warm-up jog, you'll run several times up a hill, then follow that up with a cool-down jog. On the hills, you should shorten your stride, leaning into the hill and dropping your arms so that they pump near the waist. Start conservative at the bottom of the hill and try to maintain pace the entire way up (this is Strength Work, not speed). Always "run through the hill." That is, as you approach the crest, don't slow down, but maintain your cadence even as the hill levels out. On the way down, run slowly and carefully, as injury is more likely to occur going down a hill than going up. At the bottom, jog for a minute or two before beginning the next hill climb.

TEMPO RUNS: The other cornerstone workout of the Strength Work phase, tempo runs, take a little time getting used to, but once you do, they will be an effective tool that carries over to the Track Work phase. Tempo runs are done on Tuesdays and Thursdays following your hill work weeks. On a flat, soft surface run 20 to 40 minutes at a pace that is just below your "anaerobic threshold." Simply put, run at a pace that is just below the point where you would be uncomfortable trying to hold that pace for a good length of time. This will be tricky at first, and you may go out too fast only to slow down severely after a couple minutes of running, blowing your first attempt at a tempo run. Instead, start slowly, gradually work up to a pace that is uncomfortable, then back off slightly to find tempo pace. A flat surface is key because you are getting your body to push your anaerobic threshold up by holding a pace that is just below it for a consistent amount of time—and this would be hard to do on an up-and-down course. Warm up for a mile or two before beginning a tempo run, and cool down afterward with the same distance.

THE LONG RUN: The Saturday long run carries over from the Road Work phase. If you are involved in 5K, 10K, or half-marathon training, the long run will stay constant or will vary slightly from week to week. For instance, one Saturday you might run 12 miles and the next Saturday you would run 10 miles, and then next you will run 10 miles again (for half marathon training). If you are involved in marathon training, the long run will still be building during the Strength Work phase. For instance, a Saturday long run will go from 14 miles to 18 miles in a one-week period of the Strength Work phase (marathon-training plan). Carry over all the long run lessons learned during the Road Work phase. And make sure not to skip it. The long run at this point is what gives you the endurance to handle your hill runs and your tempo runs. Without a long run for a period of weeks, you will simply "run out of gas" one day on the hills or during a tempo run. And then you will have to go back to the drawing board—back to the Road Work phase to build up your endurance again.

Note: The long run in this phase is not treated exactly the same as during the Road Work phase. You don't have two days to recover and prepare for it after the midweek run. And you don't have three days to recover from it before the midweek run. Instead, only one day separates your Thursday tempo run from your long run at the end of the week, and only two days separate your long run from your hill run on Tuesday. This means that the recovery days serve a slightly different function during the Strength Work phase (see page 17), but also the long run itself has changed. No longer is it the ultimate workout for the week—the reason for your week's running—but instead, a piece of the training week that also includes two other efforts that need to be focused on: your hill and tempo runs.

What this means physically is that the long run might have to be handled a bit gingerly in the first week or two of this phase: Start slower. Spend more time in the warm-up phase of the long run, the first couple of miles when you are getting your legs, and also resist the temptation to push it the last couple of miles.

What it also means psychologically could be just the opposite. That is, that the long run, since it is not the sole focus of the week anymore, could also become easier as the Strength Work phase goes on. There is less pressure on you to complete the long run. Instead, it is simply another workout that needs to be done during the week. Another factor making the long run easier at this point could be the fact that you are getting "more fit."

THE RECOVERY RUNS: Runners think about their upcoming runs all the time—at home, at work, during school. Whether they realize it or not, this thinking helps them get ready for the next run at hand. Yet, as any runner will tell you, there is one time when we do our best thinking about an upcoming run—and that is during a run itself, most often a run that is done the day before. Therefore, some recovery runs during the Strength Work phase take on an additional task, one that is preparatory in nature, helping you get ready for your hill workout or tempo run.

You'll do this two-for-one run by simply dividing a run in half. Spend the first 2 miles of a 4-mile run in the recovery mode—start very easy and slow down if you have to. Then shift gears and spend the next 2 miles in the preparatory mode. Freshen up the pace a little. Evaluate how you are feeling. See yourself conquering those hills or maintaining tempo pace tomorrow. You will notice the difference.

DAYS OFF: Sunday remains a day off during the Strength Work phase, but you should also consider taking some of the other recovery days off, especially in the first week or two after the shift from Road Work. For example, if the first Tuesday hill workout has really taken it out of you, come Wednesday, opt for a complete recovery day (a day off) rather than getting back out there and running. You will need to monitor your fatigue level closely at this time, because any new stress that is thrown into the training program (like the stress from a hill workout) can cause injury or illness if it is not accompanied by adequate recovery. When in doubt, take the day off.

Track Work

Track Work is where it all comes together. Road Work and Strength Work have built up to several weeks of fast running around a 400-meter oval.

What Is It?

Track Work involves 400-meter, 800-meter, 1600-meter, and 3200-meter repeats, preferably on the track, which are run once or twice a week.

What Does It Do for You?

Track Work gives you speed, the simple ability to run faster. It also helps you home in on "race pace," the tempo at which you will run all your PR-targeted races.

What Workouts Does It Include?

Track Work includes a variety of workouts at a variety of distances (400, 800, 1600, 3200 meters) on the track, plus a special workout two weeks out from your target race.

How Do I Do It?

With a sports watch, monitor your time by each lap. Workouts could be a simple collection of 400-meter repeats or something more involved like a sequence of 400s, 800s, and 1600s.

What Mental Approach Should I Take to Track Work?

Track Work is when you really have to concentrate. You'll need to focus on "exact running." That is, hitting your "splits" (the times for your intermediate distance during a repeat) so you can teach your body to run at a certain pace over a certain distance.

What Distances for Track Work Should I Expect?

Expect to run anywhere from 400 meters (a quarter of a mile) to 3200 meters (roughly two miles) at a time. During marathon training Track Work will total eight miles in one workout.

THE TRACK WORK PHASE: THE ESSENTIALS

TRACK WORK: Track Work sessions are where it all comes together in your quest to run a PR. Without Track Work, you can still race, but your races will be subpar because you won't be as fast as you truly can be. And once the gun sounds you won't have any idea of what kind of pace you are running. That's because Track Work makes you faster and helps you translate that speed into faster mile splits during your race. The overall result? You will PR. So, how do you do Track Work? It's not as simple as going down to your local high school track and running as fast as you can around it. Track Work involves a building up of speed, but also a manipulation of that speed for prime racing results.

It all starts with slow running. Each Track Work session will begin with a slow jog to warm up, followed by a set of striders to get the legs moving faster. This warm up is crucial. Without it, you run the risk of pulling a muscle or straining a tendon when you begin your first repeat on the track. And without it, the first repeats will seem monumentally hard—because you are going straight from a cold engine to a hot engine—instead of something that is moderately uncomfortable, but you can work through. Next, following the warm up, you simply need to go to the starting line with your watch set in the stopwatch mode and your workout in mind.

Here's a hint: If your track workout has more than a couple of repeats involved, divide them up into bunches. Instead of thinking about all twelve that you have to do at one time, try attacking the first four as a set, then the next four, and the final four. You can also physically divide these sets by running a double recovery after each. That is, instead of jogging 400 meters to recover after your fourth and eighth 400-meter repeat, jog 800 meters and catch your breath before diving back into the next four. Individually, each repeat (whether it is 400 meters or a mile or more) should be run as close to "even pace" as possible.

There is a big temptation to run fast at the beginning of each repeat and as you approach the end (the "breaking the tape" mentality). This should be resisted for a variety of reasons. First of all, any sudden shifts in speed can open you up to injury—a pulled muscle, a strained tendon. Also, the goal of Track Work is to help you gain familiarity through muscle memory and simple pace acumen—with your PR race pace. You do that through a series of repeats, which are run at that pace or slightly faster than this pace. Any running that is done at a pace much faster than laid out for the workout disrupts this internal monitoring process and delays you from homing in on PR race pace. Besides, the real goal of a workout like 12 x 400 meters is in accumulation. You run two, then three, then seven, then eight. And by ten, eleven, and twelve, it is a good challenge to your legs and heart and lungs to "hold pace" for the entire repeat.

If you have trouble coming in at the desired pace, you can monitor yourself early on. For instance, figure out your "split" for 200 meters of your 400-meter repeat and take a peek at your watch at this point. (It might seem awkward at first, looking down at your watch while running at a good clip, but if you simply raise the watch to your eyes rather than lowering your eyes to the watch, you will find that this motion does not interrupt your stride much and you can continue on smoothly.) Use this knowledge to either speed up or slow down your pace, remembering to stay smooth during this transition.

You'll follow each track session with a cool-down jog of a couple of miles. These can be run around the track but many find them more relaxing if they are done off the track, a signal that the "hard work" part of your workout is over. A final note to remember: Track Work is not speed work. You will be getting used to running faster than you have during your hill work and tempo runs but you won't be anywhere close to running all-out. This is because you won't ever approach that pace during your race.

THE LONG RUN: Saturdays remain a constant for the long run during the Track Work phase. For the shorter distances—5K, 10K, and half marathon—the long run will stay in a general range, varying a bit from week to week. For marathoners the long run will continue to build—18 to 20 to 22, and so on—peaking with a key long run three weeks out from race day.

At this point, during the long run, you may be tempted to run it much faster. Strength Work and now Track Work will have combined to raise your level of fitness and stimulate your fast-twitch muscle fibers. The result is that your long-run pace now seems too easy to hold for those extended miles. Should you pick up the pace and make long runs essentially an extended tempo run at this point? No. Combined with the new stress of Track Work, speeding up your long runs at this time could lead to a breakdown. Also, in speeding up your long runs—making them a tempo run—you are skipping the function of the long run at this time: to keep your level of endurance high. And without a high level of endurance, your Track Work will begin to wear you down at a time when it is most crucial—because you are approaching your race. Therefore, keep all long runs at a conversational pace during the Track Work phase.

RECOVERY RUNS: Because your fitness level is high and getting higher, you may be tempted to skip the recovery runs and perhaps squeeze in a tempo run or some other hard workout during this stage. You need to resist that temptation. And remember this: During the Track Work phase, the key workouts to target are your track workout(s), which gives you speed and pace knowledge, and your long run on Saturday, which gives you endurance. Any more hard runs during the week would be tempting fate.

DAYS OFF: Sunday will stay your day off. You might want to sleep in an extra hour to promote recovery or go for an easy walk in the afternoon to get the legs moving. But resist the temptation to make Sunday an active running day. Track Work is a jarring stress to the body and you will need at least one day a week for full recovery to keep all systems go. In fact, at this time you have the option for substituting another day off for any of your recovery runs.

How will you know when you need a day off? Generally speaking, if you wake in the morning, say, on Monday or Friday and you absolutely dread the prospect of running 4 easy miles—for physical and/or psychological reasons—maybe it is a good time to take another day off. Remember: Training is stress and then recovery. And without the needed recovery when the time comes, stress will get the better of you.

The Race-Ready Workout

To get you supremely ready to race, a Race-Ready Workout (or "secret workout") will be added to your training regime near the end of your training program. These workouts will be different depending on the race goal.

What Is It?

A Race-Ready Workout is different from the ones you have been doing in your speed phase. It will occur two or three weeks out from race day, depending on the race distance. This is enough time to let you recover and also enough time to let the "training effect" from the workout sink in.

What Does It Do for You?

It helps maximize your race readiness by giving you a very challenging— and different—workout.

What Workouts Does It Include?

Long tempo runs and "ladders," a ratcheting down of the repeat distance, while you pick up the pace. For example, for a 5K, run 1600 at 5K race pace; 1200 2 seconds faster per lap; 800 meters 4 seconds faster per lap; 400 meters 8 seconds faster per lap—with half the distance of the previous repeat as recovery.

How Do I Do It?

Run them like you would a tempo run or a hard track workout.

What Mental Approach Should I Take to the Race-Ready Workout?

You'll need to rest up in the days beforehand to be fresh for this run. You will also need to focus your utmost because no workout will prepare you for your race experience more than your race-ready run.

What Distances Should I Expect?

Distances are anywhere from a few miles of track repeats to several miles during a tempo run.

THE RACE-READY WORKOUT: THE ESSENTIALS

The Race-Ready Workout stands alone in the *How to Run a PR* process. It is not a phase that takes place over several weeks but simply a single workout, designed to efficiently prepare you for the race at hand. In this respect, outside of the race itself, it is the one running task that will matter the most to you during your sixteen weeks of training. Therefore, you need to take it seriously, making sure the recovery run the day before will put you in the right frame of mind and have your legs ready to go. You need to warm up well and follow the workout with a good cooldown and a recovery day—or two (you are going to feel more fatigued following this workout than any day since beginning the program). During the workout itself you need to resist the temptation to run it for speed, instead following the pace guidelines laid out for the workout. And you also need to give it time (don't expect to be instantly faster or more fit the following day). There is a reason it comes a good three weeks before race day: It takes time for the training effect of a hard workout to come through in actual fitness. If you have done the workout right, and we have timed it right, that fitness should come through for you at a crucial time: on race day.

Some Other Training Philosophies

The program components I've just described—Road, Strength, Track, Race-Ready—do not make for the only running program out there (but we think it is the best for most runners). Here's a quick look at some other possible programs you might have encountered when you were searching for ways in which to PR.

THE ALL-DISTANCE PLAN

This plan has you running exclusively long, slow distance. All the runs are easy, at a conversational pace, and you gradually up your mileage from week to week to achieve a heightened level of fitness. Probably the most used program among beginning level runners who are training to race.

PROS: It's easy. Chance of injury is low. You will raise your level of endurance.

CONS: Speed stays stagnant. Or just inches up. There are no targeted workouts to home in on race pace.

THE ALL-SPEED PLAN

This plan has you running almost exclusively speed workouts during the week. All the runs are fast, mainly on the track, and you begin the program running, say, 400 meter repeats at a certain pace, and end the program running them at a much faster pace. This program was used a lot several decades ago and still has some adherents today.

PROS: You will get faster. And you stand a good chance at homing in on race pace.

CONS: You can't stay with it for long. Chance of burnout or injury is very high.

SPEED FIRST, DISTANCE LATER

This plan has you running several weeks of speed workouts on the track, then shifting over to several weeks of long, slow distance off the track. It is used to get the legs moving fast right away.

PROS: You get a good mix, and you will be able to run your long runs at a faster pace.

CONS: Distance comes at a time when you need to be concentrating on pace work for your upcoming race. There is also a high danger of injury when beginning with speed.

DISTANCE, SPEED, DISTANCE

This plan has you building up with long, slow distance work, then shifting over to several weeks of speed, before shifting back to distance to work on the well of endurance before the race. Used mainly for the half marathon and the full marathon.

PROS: You will be able to cover the distance.

CONS: There is a danger of slowing down, falling off pace, just when you need to focus on speed in your training.

CHAPTER 4

Other Things You Need to Know to PR

This book covers training for a PR in chapters and training schedules; it also covers race week in a separate chapter. But there are several other things that can influence your pursuit of a PR, and the more you know about them, the more likely you will be able to make your PR quest a success. This chapter contains a discussion of several topics, all of which are essential to your PR quest.

When to Train

Picking the right time of year to go after a PR is crucial in determining your success. Except for those who live in the Southwest or Deep South, most of us would not expect to PR during the months of December, January, or February (it would be much too cold, snowy, windy, and icy to navigate a fast time during these months).

But many runners still chase PRs during the summer months of June, July, and August. Summer is a tempting time of year to chase a PR. The sun is shining. You can train in the bare essentials, making you feel fast and loose. The paths and roads and tracks are filled with fellow runners, giving you a sense that this, indeed, is the season for running. Plus, if your PR quest involves a 5K or 10K, you don't have to wait around long—there is a race (or two or three) just about every weekend, so if you come up short one weekend, you just have to wait around seven days for another chance. What better time to turn your attention to racing, right?

Wrong. As tempting as it is to jump on the racing bandwagon during the summer, if you are serious about setting a PR to be proud of—if you want to see just how fast you can really run for a 5K, 10K, half marathon, or marathon—you don't want to answer the starting gun in June, July, or August. Why? The simple answer is that it is too hot—too hot to race in.

Most marathons—the ultimate test for you as a runner—take place during the spring and fall. During those seasons, the weather is cool enough that everyone can run well. Granted, as the race distance goes down, heat becomes less a factor (because you are not out there battling the heat for as long) until you get to the sprints (100, 200, and 400 meters) where runners actually like the temperatures to be in the 70s or above. But generally speaking, any race where the temperatures start inching up above the low 60s, is a race where 99.9 percent of all runners are not going to be able to race at their highest levels. Why is that? The simple explanation is that in hotter weather you have to work harder to keep going at the same pace. You will breathe faster, your heart will race faster, you will sweat. This "uncomfortable reality" will cause you to either slow down dramatically or to ratchet down your race pace before you even begin.

To better your chances at reaching a PR, target races in the spring and fall. Aim your four months of training so that they will culminate (with a singular race like the marathon or a series of shorter races if you are targeting the 5K and 10K) in the spring or fall. By doing that you are almost guaranteeing yourself ideal temperatures for your race-day quest.

Ideal weather for your PR might not be exactly what you think it should be. Most runners will do better in slightly—or even more severely—colder weather, such as the mid-50s or even high 40s. Once you get going, and your body heats up with the effort of the race, you will find that the coldness has disappeared. Instead, the coldness has been replaced by an invigorating little bite in the air. That little bite in the air, coupled with the fact that you are running through "neutral weather" (it is neither too hot for the body nor too cold) helps you get "in the zone."

There will be a further discussion of this concept in Chapter 6 for when you are getting ready to race but for now we can say that being "in the zone" is when you are nailing race pace, when the miles click by with a strange combination of heavy effort and comfort. Getting in the zone—and staying in it—requires supreme focus and concentration, and this is easier to do when you feel a little invigorating bite in the air along your fingertips.

A final note: Some runners claim to be "hot weather runners" and they can point to the fact that they have run their best races—their PRs—during the summer months when temperatures have been 80 degrees or above. This may be so, but there are two possible explanations for this: (1) They are the exceptions to the rule. (2) They have never really tested themselves by training for, and racing in, a spring or fall race. Instead, they simply run through those months, waiting for the summer months to come around again. These people may have convinced themselves that they are "hot weather runners" but they will never know their actual PRs.

Shoes

You cannot possibly set a PR training in an old pair of shoes, so the first thing you need to do before you begin a training program is examine your shoes.

- Are the treads in the soles worn smooth?
- Is the heel counter crushed or broken down?
- Are the laces broken and retied to keep them together?
- If so, pick up that pair and throw them in your trash can.

Even if your shoes exhibit none of the above, they could still be way past the point of no return, the point where they are no longer cushioning your footfall, springing you back, and helping you move on down the road. (That's because shoes break down internally before externally.)

How do you know when your shoes have reached this point? Many runners keep track of the mileage on their shoes or date them to know when it is time to purchase new shoes. But running in a pair of shoes for an arbitrary number of miles or number of months is only a general rule that could lead to decreased training or injury.

The best way to know if it is time for new shoes is to know you: Are you feeling flat for several days in a row? Are your knees aching a little after each run? Do you have the sensation when running of your feet "sticking" to the ground?

If so, you need to get a new pair of running shoes.

And when you are at the running shoe store, you might consider getting a second pair of the same shoes so that you can "rotate" shoes while training. Rotating shoes (you wear the first pair on Monday, the second pair on Tuesday, and the first pair on Wednesday, etc.) was first devised as a way to make your running shoes last longer. The thinking was that a single pair of shoes would get a rest between runs, since you were not running in the same pair each day, and that during that rest period the internal cushioning of the shoes would have a chance to spring back and recover, rather than continually be crushed and pounded by your footfalls, and therefore, your shoes would last longer.

Whether rotating shoes actually helps your shoes last longer is still up for debate. But what is not debatable is this: Rotating your shoes will ensure that your shoes are not broken down a few months into training program as you have been training on two pairs, not one.

Stretching

Stretching becomes very important during the Strength Work and Track Work phases of your PR training program—when you are really stretching out your legs—but don't wait until you begin your Strength Work to begin a stretching program. A good time to start incorporating stretching is during the first weeks of your Road Work phase. This will do two things: prevent your legs from "locking up" during all that long, slow distance (which you will cover in short strides) and keep your legs "open" for hill running and thus avoid early strains and pulls when you start heading up the hills.

Two or three times a week—following a recovery run—devote 10 minutes to some easy stretching. (Note: Don't stretch after any of your hard workouts for the week—the long run, midweek run, hill work, tempo runs, or track work. That is when the leg muscles will be tired and most susceptible to strains or tears.)

Here are six stretches designed to get you ready to PR:

THE HAMSTRING STRETCH: Place one leg up on a park bench or chair with the knee as straight as you can get it. With the other leg straight, bend forward at the waist and lean through the leg that is up on the bench or chair. The hamstring is the large muscle on the back of the upper leg. You should feel a good stretch. Hold for 20 seconds. Relax and repeat with the other leg. Do two sets.

THE CALF STRETCH: Stand two feet from a wall and place both hands on the wall, then drop one leg back behind you, keeping that knee locked and that foot flat on the floor. Feel the stretch in the calf muscle—the large muscle behind the leg between the ankle and the knee—by leaning into the wall. Hold for 20 seconds. Relax and repeat with the other leg. Do two sets.

THE QUADRICEPS STRETCH: With your left hand braced against the back of a park bench or a solid object, grab the front of your right ankle with your right hand and pull your heel to your butt, feeling the stretch in your right "quad"—the large muscle in front of the leg between the knee and the hip. Hold for 20 seconds. Relax and repeat with the other leg. Do two sets. (Note: Stand tall with your back straight during this stretch to maximize its effectiveness.)

THE SOLEUS STRETCH: Stand six inches away from a wall with both hands on the wall and all your weight on one leg. Bend that knee and angle your weight into the wall, feeling the stretch in the soleus muscle—the muscle at the base of the back of the leg, just above the Achilles tendon. Hold for 20 seconds. Relax and repeat with the other leg. Do two sets. (Note: Be very gentle with this stretch the first time out. The soleus can be sensitive.)

THE GROIN STRETCH: Stand straight with your legs wide apart. Bend the right knee and bend your torso over that knee, keeping your left leg straight and your left foot flat on the ground, feeling the stretch along the left side of the groin—the area at the top inside of your leg. Hold for 20 seconds. Relax and repeat with the other leg. Do two sets.

THE TRUNK STRETCH: Lie flat on your back with both knees bent and your arms out perpendicular and straight. Gently roll both knees to the right side of your body while turning your head to the left side, feeling the stretch all through the right side of your trunk—the large muscles in your back and side between your chest and waist. Hold for 20 seconds. Relax and repeat with the opposite side. Do two sets.

Note: After two weeks of these stretches, increase the duration of each stretch by 10 seconds to 30 seconds. Two weeks later, increase the duration another 10 seconds to 40 seconds. Keep progressing until you are stretching for a minute each time. Also make sure you are not "forcing the stretch" (where real pain comes into the stretch), which can tear muscle fiber instead of stretching it.

Overtraining

Overtraining generally strikes high school or college level runners who are racing a lot and trying to squeeze high-quality runs in among those races, but it can also become a burden for the recreational runner, especially those who have embarked upon an ambitious training regime, like one you would follow to run a PR.

For our purposes, overtraining is a gradual—or sometimes sudden—wearing out of the body because you have been training too much (in the Road Work phase) or too hard (in the Strength Work or Track Work phases). Or both. If overtraining is not monitored and nipped in the bud, you will find yourself in need of several weeks or more of rest to bounce back, and therefore unable to continue with the PR training program you set out for yourself.

So how do we know if we are overtrained? Overtraining is tricky. Sometimes it is hard to distinguish from simple fatigue—the body will be tired the following day from, say, a Saturday long run or a Tuesday hill workout. But generally, any fatigue that lingers through the week and into the next, can be a sign that you are overtrained. A morning resting heartbeat that is above normal for several days in a row and a sudden loss of a couple of pounds or more can be signs. Notice as well any disruptions in your normal sleep patterns; for example, you find it nearly impossible to get out of bed in the morning or you wake up continuously throughout the night (the body is too tired even to get good rest)—these are also associated with overtraining. In terms of training, you may no longer look forward to running and a workout as simple as a 4-mile recovery run becomes something to "be endured," and early in your runs you have thoughts of packing it in.

Overtrained? Take the Coffee Test

Overtraining affects all parts of your body, not just your legs. One of the first cues that you are overtraining, or on the verge of overtraining, is that your nerves are on edge. A good way to gauge this is to take the coffee test. A good cup of coffee in the morning should perk you up, not set you on edge (that usually happens after several cups). If your first cup in the morning makes you grind your teeth, you could be overtraining.

When you're training for a PR, you may experience overtraining for several reasons:

Your body is not yet ready to handle the workload it has been given. You are following a training schedule that the body is not recovering from. It is breaking down instead.

If this is you, you can still salvage your race goals by taking some time off to try and snap yourself out of the overtrained mode. Try running short and slow for a week. Or simply take three days off in a row, concentrating on getting plenty of sleep. Then when you start back with your regular training schedule, add an additional day off to your week—make it one of the recovery days. Many times that is all you need.

You're not putting enough emphasis on rest days and recovery days. Those days should all be easy days (and with the rest day, a complete day off). Some runners feel they are strong enough to turn some—or all—of those days into quality workouts. For instance, the Monday recovery run of 4 miles becomes 8 miles because 8 miles is more of a workout than 4 (or a fast 4 miles supplants a slow 4 miles because you can only get faster by running fast, right?). The end result is that without adequate rest and recovery days the body simply becomes overwhelmed by all the stress. (Even elite marathoners divide their weekly workouts between those that will stress the body and those that are designed to help the body recover from that stress, and rarely do the stress-inducing days number more than three per week.)

If you've been disregarding your easy days, you need to immediately emphasize your rest, recovery, and preparatory days. Put your feet up on your day off and start slow and stay slow during your recovery and preparatory runs. Most of the time, this will get you back where you need to be—fresh and ready for your hard workouts.

You set the bar too high. This kind of overtraining is particular to the Track Work phase, and has to do with the body not accepting the pace with which the track workouts are run. In short, you are training so fast—the 400s, 800s, and miles—that every workout becomes a race (something that is breaking you down), rather than a controlled workout that is teaching you pace (something that you can build on).

If this is the case—you have set a PR goal that is too ambitious, and the Track Work you are running to attain that goal is wearing you out—you can still salvage your quest by swallowing your pride and doing one thing: Training for a less ambitious PR. You can do this by simply picking the next training program in the book (one that is slower) and follow that instead. For instance, Track Work for a 25-minute 5K is causing you to overtrain. Skip to the 27:30 program and see if that is a better fit for you.

You skipped part of the Road Work phase. There is no quicker way to sink into an overtraining hole than to pile on hill work or tempo runs or Track Work without first adding a base of miles to your training through Road Work. The long, slow miles you put in for weeks during the Road Work phase help the body endure the stress of those workouts. Without it, you are training on borrowed time.

If you have skipped all or most of your Road Work phase—you have my sympathy. There is really nothing you can do but get a few good weeks of complete rest, then go back to the drawing board—go back and put in the weeks of Road Work that you neglected. In other words, you have to start this program all over again.

Undertraining

The opposite of overtraining, undertraining, will become apparent in the first week of the Track Work phase of the PR training program. You may find yourself, even from day one, way ahead of the curve because your Road Work and Strength Work have given you a level of fitness far beyond that which you predicted at the start of the program. The end result is that by the time you get to Track Work, the pace at which you're running your 400s or 800s or miles (to nail that pace for your 10K) is not even winding you. And when you finish the requisite number of repeats, you can still go on and do more, sometimes much more. What has happened is that neither the speed nor the volume of Track Work is stressing you. Your Track Work, then, is a simple going through the motions, an attempt to teach your body to race at a pace that it can already hold quite comfortably.

What you need to do in this instance is first of all recognize undertraining early in the Track Work phase. And this might be harder than it seems. The temptation here will be to simply bask in your fitness—look at me, I can do all my workouts with ease—not realizing that the end result is a squandering of fitness, because you never took it to the next level.

And the next level is what you are after. If you realize you are undertraining, you need to adjust your PR time goal to something faster. Track Work takes eight weeks to finish. If you can identify undertraining in the first week and make that adjustment, you will have seven weeks of solid workouts at your new goal pace. Enough time to race at a higher level.

Injury Prevention

Getting to the starting line healthy is of maximum importance for your PR. A nagging injury can be the difference between nailing that PR and coming home seconds short. Along with stretching, there are several preventive measures you can take to keep injuries at bay while training for your PR:

• **Never replace your rest and recovery days with hard workouts.** There are two times when the temptation will be the strongest to replace your rest and recovery days with hard workouts. The first is midway through your Road Work phase when your endurance level is rising and the Sunday morning following your long run you feel the urge to get out and do it again. The second time is during your Track Work phase when you can feel yourself getting more "race ready" by the week and the urge to "hit the oval" for an unscheduled workout is strong. These temptations must be resisted as you remember that without adequate rest and recovery, all the stress of hard running will gang up on you.

- **Always run in newish shoes.** As discussed earlier, you should begin the training programs in this book with shoes no more than a couple of weeks old (and preferably rotate pairs).

- **Avoid running on concrete.** Concrete bounces most of the force of each stride back up into the legs and body, making it a poisonous surface to run on. Ideal surfaces for key workouts are as follows: a soft jogging path or trail for all long runs, tempo runs, and recovery runs; and a cushioned track for all Track Work. Hill work will be tricky. It might be impossible to find a good hill that is not on a road (though you should try to find one at your area parks). If you need to run a hill workout on a road out of necessity, try to find a road that is made of asphalt, not concrete.

- **Start slow.** Any sudden shift in speed—particularly one that comes at the beginning of a workout—can cause a pulled muscle or muscle strain. For hill runs, that means you should "wind into" the hill, jogging slower, then faster, as you approach the bottom of the hill, working up to the pace at which you want to run. For tempo runs, that means you should work up to tempo pace after a couple hundred yards or so of running. For Track Work, that means you should use the distance from the start to the first curve to "find pace," rather than attempting to immediately be there when you start your watch.

- **End controlled.** The final straight on the track during your last repeat, cresting the hill for the last hill climb, the last minute of a tempo run, the last half mile of a long run—these are all instances when the temptation to finish really fast will be strong. Yet you need to remember that any sudden shift in speed, especially in these instances—when you are tired from a long, hard workout that is coming to an end—could cause injury. Instead, remind yourself here that the goal of each hard workout is to complete it in one piece.

• **Avoid the stairs.** On the days that your legs are sore from the previous day's hard workout, take the escalator or elevator, not the stairs. Climbing up—and especially going down—puts unnatural stress on your knees and hips and could lead to one of those little annoyance injuries that blossom into something much more severe.

• **Sleep.** A tired body is more prone to injury than an awake, alert body. (Just the fact that you are tired means that you are not fully recovered and that the body has not fully repaired itself.) During your PR training, try for eight to nine hours of sleep each night. And on the weekends, squeeze in a nap Saturday afternoon following your long run and another on Sunday afternoon during your day off.

Training Partners

There will be days when no one can meet you to run. And there will be days when you don't want to run with anyone else—when an easy 4 miles by yourself on a park trail is just what you need. But for the most part, you should map out your PR training program, a program that takes four months to complete, by scheduling runs with others. It could be the difference between nailing that PR—or not.

Why? There are no scientific studies to back this up, but running with a training partner or a group makes it easier to complete your run. Simply put, less effort has to be expended mentally and physically. Elite athletes have known this for ages. That is why you will always see packs of runners early on in major marathons. They have bunched together purposely: to help each other out.

So, on a day when you are scheduled to complete a 14-mile long run (and are feeling kind of crappy) or a day when you are scheduled to do a long series of hill climbs (and are feeling kind of crappy), having one or more human beings alongside will be the tonic you need to complete them, rather than stop your workout short.

Training partners do more than just run alongside you in a sort of moving comfort. They also provide moral support. If you are going through some rough patches in your training, having a day or a week when you just don't feel 100 percent, it can help to have another runner to discuss it with (especially during a run) and keep you going in the right direction.

Training partners also keep you consistent. You will be running five or six times a week for 16 weeks in the PR Training Program. That's a lot of running you have to look forward to—or not. Knowing that you are meeting a training partner for a run will keep you on schedule, especially on those days when you just don't feel like it.

So, what makes for a good training partner?

The first quality you should look for in a training partner is mutual speed. The reason for this is obvious. All your workouts—long runs, easy runs, hill runs, tempo runs, Track Work—can be done together, in virtual lockstep (some days you may be faster, and some days your training partner may be a bit faster, but that only helps keep it interesting). And if you have similar racing goals—say, you are both going after a 1:50 PR in the half marathon this fall—then you can race together as well as train together.

That said, you can still benefit from a training partner who is slower or faster than you. Agree to meet during mutual recovery days, when you both are running easy. You can do these runs together. Long runs are a different animal. Unless the faster runner agrees to slow down for the slower runner, you will inevitably finish far apart. Yet some mutual benefit can be gained simply by starting together and knowing that you are not alone. This concept is perhaps more noticeable during Strength Work and Track Work. Doing these runs with runners who are faster or slower than you will not provide any immediate help in terms of pacing. But starting together, finishing while others are at the finish line or at the top of the hill, and simply being out there together—pushing it hard, while others around you are doing the same—will have a positive effect on your training.

The second quality you should look for is punctuality. Having a training partner who consistently shows up 15 or 20 minutes late for a run is like having no training partner at all (you are long gone by that time). We all have lives outside of running and many times we are squeezing in our runs around those lives. A good training partner realizes this and respects the beginning time of each run.

The third quality is a bit harder to get a handle on, but a good training partner should either be a good friend or have the potential to become one. You can only talk about running for so long, so you need to have mutual interests to pass the time during long runs. You also need someone to commiserate with if your workouts have not been going as well as planned. And you need someone to pump you up in those last few weeks before race time.

You can find plenty of training partners by joining a local running club and participating in their group runs. Inevitably, though, you should pair off, picking one from that large group (with the qualities above) to become your individual training partner.

CHAPTER 5

More Things You Need to Know to PR

There are still more things you need to know to PR. We continue with that discussion in this chapter.

A Smallish Race

You stand a better chance of nailing your PR if you enter a race where you don't have to fight through crowds of other runners in the opening miles—or all the way to the finish line. Generally speaking, the longer the race, the more people that can be entered and still have the race course conducive to a PR. That means for a marathon or half marathon, a couple thousand people entered in the race should be a limit. For 5Ks and 10Ks, try to pick a race that has an entry field in the hundreds, not the thousands.

And just as you don't want too many runners in your race, you don't want too few. Entering a half marathon that has thirty-six runners in an effort to PR will just make it harder on you. You will find yourself running alone for much of the race, instead of around a group of runners who may be running at a similar pace and who can help make your PR quest easier.

So how do you find out where and when the small races will occur? Ask your fellow runners. Contact a running club. Check out race websites for information on race size, or simply call the race ahead of time and ask.

A GOOD RACE COURSE

Picture this: You are approaching mile 4 of your 10K. The first 3 miles have gone like clockwork, you are feeling great, right on pace, and can almost taste that PR. Then you turn a corner on the race course and there in front of you is a hill about as steep as the one you used to sled down as a kid—and twice as long.

By the time you get to the top of it, running a PR that day is a distant dream.

Unless you are in much better shape than you think you are, then you are probably not going to PR on a hilly race course. Going up those hills will slow your pace down and keep you from reaching your PR goals. Similarly, a country 10K, where 5 miles of the race are run on a rocky, pitted, dirt road, is not going to be conducive to a PR, either. Your stride will be slipping on the uneven surface, making it much harder to hold your race pace.

Like the homework you did to find out the size of a possible race you might enter, you also need to do some homework to figure out the lay of the land. Talk with fellow runners and running club officials, and contact race directors to find out about possible PR pitfalls, like big hills, uneven race surfaces, wind off the lake, even an abundance of turns. And if a race you have been considering running is plagued with one or more of these maladies, cross it off your race schedule and look for another.

This might sound like nitpicking, but if you come up seven seconds short in your PR quest on a course where the wind off the lake was blowing into your body like a hand on your chest during the last mile, you will wake up the next morning thinking about a lost opportunity: "If only the wind hadn't kicked up. . . ."

A good race course, first and foremost, needs to be flat. This doesn't mean it has to be pool-table flat the entire way, but for the most part, the course shouldn't have any grades where you need to put your head down and work to get to the top. A flat course will give you the best chance to get on pace and stay on pace the entire race distance, and you should look for this in a 5K or 10K race course.

That said, gentle, rolling hills can actually help during a longer race. Such hills can tax the leg muscles in a slightly different way than all that flat running, giving some muscles a break. And they provide a minibreak for the mind as well, taking it off cruise control, which it turned on during the monotony of all those long, flat miles.

The second thing you need to look for in a good race course is the surface. Ideally, the surface beneath your feet should be paved. This will ensure a solid footfall and push off with each and every stride. Park paths and canal towpaths and the like are great places to train—the soft dirt surface limits pounding on the legs, and you can recover from a long run on a path much sooner than the roads—but when your foot hits this surface it is slipping a little with each stride. The end result is you are not as efficient a racer on a path as you would be on a road.

As far as what surface your road should be, for the most part, it should be asphalt. This is not a hard and fast rule. You can get away with racing a 5K and 10K on concrete, which is a fast surface. But generally, as your race distance gets longer—half marathons and marathons—you should be looking at a race course that is mainly asphalt, a much softer surface than concrete, to save your legs, because in those races the later miles essentially become a battle between you and sore legs. The more sore your legs are at that point, the more likely you are to slow down and fall off pace.

The third thing you should look for is something I will call "enclosure." This concept has to do with the fact that it is generally harder to run through a wide open space than in an environment that has a sense of closeness. Certain running tracks in Europe are known as fast, precisely because they are enclosed to a degree that makes them more intimate than the big stadiums. Just take a run down an open, deserted road to see what I am talking about. Then take the same distance run through a tree-lined neighborhood.

The second venue should be an easier place to run precisely because the distance gets lost in the environment, rather than emphasized by the open road. Therefore as a general PR guideline, look for a race course that is urban, as opposed to one that is out in the wide open country.

The Track

For the most part, the boom in jogging paths in the 1990s was good for the sport. It cut running injuries in half (because the paths were much softer than roads and sidewalks) and it got people to run through nature as opposed to running through traffic. Yet it did one thing that was detrimental to the sport: It kept runners away from the running track.

I'm not talking about casual joggers, who opted to run their 4 miles on a park path, as opposed to doing 16 laps around the track (who wouldn't make that choice?). And I'm not talking about the hard-core racer who took to the jogging path for the majority of his runs but returned to the track for his weekly speed work.

I am talking about the new runner-turned-racer who found the sport on the jogging paths and refused to leave it, running all her workouts—slow or fast—on the same 4-mile loop or 6-mile out-and-back course that saw her baptism into the sport. These runners may have been running hard when they did their faster-paced work on the trail on Tuesdays, and they still may have been racing well on Saturdays. But they were selling themselves short by refusing to hit the track.

"The Track" is a mysterious, intimidating place for runners who have never been there before: A 400-meter oval with two long straight aways, two curves, often behind a fence that is locked to the public. Many new runners shy away from the track because of what it seems to represent—hard, fast, brutal running that is more pain than gain and will leave them bent double and gasping for breath. Yet doing key workouts on the track is vital to the success of your PR quest.

For starters, the track is expertly measured and marked. To run a PR it is imperative that you have "innate pace knowledge," that is, a built-in monitoring system that lets you know when you are running on race pace and when you are not. The best way to get innate pace knowledge is through repetition, say, a series of 400s, or 800s, or miles on a flat course where you are assured of the distance you are running. On a track, you can monitor your pace as early as half a lap around (an eighth of a mile) and continue making adjustments every 200 meters if you wish. Try doing this on a jogging path whose only markers are one per mile.

The track is also precise. One lap is the same as the next, is the same as the next, is the same as the next, making an even, on-pace effort pay off. This will not always be true on a jogging path or road, where perhaps variations in the terrain can make the second 400-meter segment of a repeat 800 meters harder than the previous one. Running a workout on a course like this will miss the point of the workout (to have your body do a series of repeats at a certain pace and learn the effort it takes to run that pace) because this will cause you to either fall off pace for your workout or to put much more effort than is normal into your run up a short hill, say, for you to stay on pace.

Finally, the track will make you faster. I'm not simply talking about the result of doing all those workouts on the track, which will surely make you faster. What I'm talking about occurs the first time you set foot on a track. You will feel it almost instantaneously. The track is not a jogging path or a sidewalk. The track is serious. It has lanes, a starting line and a finish line. It is designed for competition, a place where runners give 100 percent of their effort to round that last turn and head for home. This can be intimidating at first, and the reason why many runners over the years have refused to set foot on a track. Yet the key to running any workout on a track is to harness that energy, that excitement. And if you can do that, you will take your faster-paced workouts to a new level. Think about it: If Track Work can squeeze just one second out of you per 400 meters, that's 4 seconds for every mile. Translate that to a 10K, and you have run 25 seconds faster for your race!

How to Run on the Track

- **Warm Up and Cool Down Off the Track.** If your workout calls for a 1- or 2-mile jog to warm up and a 1- or 2-mile jog to cool down, run these off the track. The reason for this is twofold: First of all, jogging on a track is boring. You don't want to lose enthusiasm for your workout before it has begun. Second, you want to keep the track a sacred place. By this I mean you want to let your body know that each and every time you step on the track, you will be doing a run that taxes the body, hard work. By making sure to warm up and cool down off the track, you are reinforcing this concept.

- **Take the Inside Lane.** The track is measured from the inside of lane one. Running in lane two or veering off into lane three on the curve will make you run farther.

- **Don't Sprint for Home.** We've all seen exciting finishes in track meets on TV. But when you are running repeat 400s, 800s, and miles, you are after an even pace the entire way. That means holding effort on the final turn. That means no sprint finishes. As we've discussed earlier, sprinting to the finish line is a good way to pull a muscle and end your quest for a PR.

- **Find Your Time to Run.** At certain times of day—late afternoon, most likely—the track can be crowded with a high school or college team that is having a practice. Find a time on the track that is yours. This could mean an early morning trek to the track or maybe one at lunchtime or in the evening. Each track will be different, so you might want to look at one or two in your area before making a decision about which track to call home. (Also, don't be afraid to drive to a track, like you would a running path. Park and then run.)

Staying Smooth

If you have ever been to a race, you have heard this phrase, "stay smooth," repeated a number of times to a number of runners as they battled through a midrace stretch or homed in on the finish. Once the gun sounds, staying smooth is perhaps the number one key to notching that PR. But what does it mean? Essentially, "staying smooth" means running with a lack of tension in the body, and it is easier said than done. This is because as we get tired from continued running, all of us inevitably begin to tense up, and this in turn causes us to slow down by shortening our stride or slowing our cadence or both.

Ideally, then, you want to stay smooth—avoid tension—for as long as possible. You can do this by starting slow, staying slow, and finishing slow (but that won't get you a PR). Or you can race like you mean it, and use these tips to help you stay smooth during your race:

- Keep your head up or tilted slightly forward. You want to avoid a backward lean of your head.
- Keep your eyes focused forward, down the road. Not to the side or—definitely not—behind you. This will cause you to turn your head around, which will cause tension.
- Keep your jaw loose, not clenched. A loose lower lip can do the trick.
- Keep your shoulders slightly leaning forward and down. Raising your shoulders can lock up the upper body.
- Keep your elbows loose.
- Don't clench your fists (even when you are driving for the finish line). Hold your hands in a loose fist, as if you are holding a small bird. Keep your thumbs out but not pointed up.
- Keep your torso loose, not rigid. It shouldn't feel locked to the hips.
- Keep the hips loose. They should feel like they are riding above the legs, not attached to them.
- If you need to change your stride pattern, shorten your stride and concentrate on upping your cadence, rather than lengthening your stride, which can lock up your legs and slow you down.
- Concentrate on getting your knees up and out, not simply up.
- Keep landing midfoot, not on your toes or heel.
- Wiggle your toes inside your shoes. Really. If you can do this, you are loose.

Note: Within the basic framework of the running stride, we all have our own peculiarities. For example, John's left arm comes out a little more than usual; Julie leans forward more than most; or Dick has a short, choppy stride. These differences from the norm—the textbook stride—have been engrained in us over time because it was the way we adapted to the exercise, the way we could get down that road most efficiently because, hey, that was—is—who we are. Staying smooth has nothing to do with correcting these peculiarities. What staying smooth has to do with is keeping your basic stride—whether it is shortish or leaning forward or uses an exaggerated arm swing—for as long as possible during your race.

A Good Running Watch

A good running watch is a very important piece of equipment for your PR quest. It is essential for several workouts, which I shall get to in a moment. For now, let's go over what a good sports watch has to have:

• A stopwatch function. That is, a mode that gives you a running clock (in seconds and minutes) from the time you start it to the time you stop it. When the stopwatch function is on, the face should be easy to read when held at waist level. This is very important because during Track Work you want to keep your stride as fluid as possible, and raising your wrist to your face to squint at your splits (your intermediate times, like your 400-meter times during a fast mile) until they come into focus will cause your run to be jerky and unbalanced. (Most people will slow down to see their splits, then jerk back into a faster running pace once they have lowered their arms.)

• "Start," "stop," and "reset" buttons that are easy to press and—this is important—that respond easily. There is nothing more aggravating during a run than to look down at your stopwatch and see that the time you have spent running is 00:00 because the stopwatch did not start when you pressed it. (For this reason many runners have a conditioned double take when starting their stopwatch function at the beginning of their runs. The second take is to make sure the stopwatch started.)

• A comfortable wristband, one that does not bite or twist or pull. If there is a big difference between the holes (one is too tight and the other is too loose), consider getting another watch or at least shopping around for another band. (The only thing more aggravating while running than having your watch flop around on your wrist is having your watch band around your wrist like a noose.)

Once you have a good running watch, you'll want to put it to use. You will use your watch for a variety of functions during a variety of workouts. Let's take them one at a time:

• **The long run:** Even though your goal for a long run is a certain number of miles, time all your long runs with your stopwatch function. This is important because you will need a first-mile split to make sure you are going slow enough, and maybe a midrace pace check, too, if you are running a route where you have measured miles. Make sure to keep the time running during your long run because, late in the run, looking at your watch and seeing the accumulated time that you have run (an hour, an hour and a half, two hours) can act as a boost of confidence at that point, just when you might be feeling like packing it in.

• **The tempo run:** The key to executing a good tempo run is to find your pace early by referring to your watch at the half-mile or mile point, locking into that pace, and then forgetting about your watch for a while. You will need your watch, however, to signal the end of the tempo run (you will have to use your internal clock to know when to take a peek) or you may just stretch this workout into something more stressful than it was meant to be.

- **Track Work:** The watch is the tale of the tape for all your track workouts. But you need to know how to use your watch efficiently. Practice a "rolling start." You should be able to click your watch to start the stopwatch mode at the same time as you are beginning to run quickly. This will make your track repeats go smoother, eliminating the cold start, where you start the stopwatch as you are standing still, then, sprint out to make up for that lost second. Similarly, you might need to go over your finish once or twice. Ideally, you should be able to hold form and pace through the finish line while simply reaching over with your right hand to stop the stopwatch function on your left wrist. Also, resist the temptation to peek at your watch constantly, most notably on your final lap or as you approach the finish line. Instead, run through the finish. Jog for a step or two. Then look at your watch for your time. You might be happily surprised at the results. (Don't let your watch take over your Track Workouts. The stopwatch is the gauge you will use to measure your workout but the purpose of the workout is to get yourself used to running a certain pace for a certain distance. This will happen much more slowly—or it might not happen at all—if you are interrupting your run all the time to look at your watch.)

- **Recovery runs:** An often forgotten tool here, but your stopwatch function is vital during recovery runs because, like the long run, the watch can be used to make sure you are running slowly enough early in your run by getting a time for the first mile. Also, a look at your total time at the end of a recovery run reinforces the fact that you have run little that day and have recovered.

- **Visualization days:** As your race day approaches, you might find this little trick to be of help in getting you prepared for the race at hand. When you have some time, start your watch and let it run out to your exact PR goal time (for example, 50:00 for a 10K), then stop the watch there. Carry that time around with you on your stopwatch and refer to it often during the day for some mini-motivation.

Nutrition

If there is one thing that's a constant in terms of runners and their diets, it's that there is no such thing as the ideal runner's diet. Everyone is different. For example, many runners focus on pasta to get their carbs, while others make rice their main carbohydrates; still others load up on bread. I have known runners who seemingly eat nothing but chocolate, and others who swear off sweets. I have also known some road race champions who are strict vegetarians and others who like a good steak. I know runners who drink a lot of milk and others who let nothing but fruit juice and/or water pass through their lips.

Yet, at a certain point in our running lives, our runner's diet becomes like our stride pattern—we have developed one that works best for us. And I am guessing that most of you reading this book have already reached that point. You have found that the handful of peanuts gulped midafternoon gets you through your late afternoon run, and that Chinese food on Saturday nights is a good way for you to recover from your Saturday morning long run (you can feel the recovery working as you wake on Sunday morning). Therefore, to change your diet at this point would be counterproductive. To change it while training for a PR, in fact, could cause you to fail by adding stress to your training week. Food should not cause stress. Food is there for energy and recovery.

That said, here are a few general eating guidelines to follow while you are training for your PR:

• **Pump up the carbs:** Carbohydrate is your energy source for most of the running you will be doing, and to fall into carbohydrate debt will cause your energy levels to plummet and your workouts to suffer. How do you keep from falling into a carbohydrate debt? Simply make sure that you are eating some carbohydrates with every meal and supplement your meals following a hard workout—long run, tempo run, hill run, Track Work—with extra carbs, like another piece of bread, a second helping of potatoes, or a carbohydrate-rich energy drink during the day.

• **Don't skip breakfast:** A key to working out consistently during your quest for a PR is consistent energy levels. You accomplish this by training smartly, resting wisely—and by eating breakfast. Nothing damages your daily energy level more than skipping breakfast. It is at breakfast time when your body and your mind are most hungry—you haven't eaten for more than eight hours. It is also at breakfast time when you need to eat to energize your workout later in the day. A bowl of cereal, toast with a smear of peanut butter, and a glass of orange juice at 7:30 a.m. is really your key meal for your 5:30 p.m. mile repeats on the track.

• **Snack:** Another way to keep energy levels consistent during the long grind of the training process is to snack. Something as simple as a mid-morning apple (not two doughnuts) can boost energy levels and also ensure that you won't be overeating for lunch. Snack times are midmorning, late afternoon, and, for some, late at night (which is a good time to get in some extra carbs if you feel you might be deficient). The key to snacking is also the key to your meals: Make it healthy and make it light. For example, a small bag of pretzels late in the afternoon would be preferable over a cherry Danish. But if you are going to eat an entire large bag of pretzels you might as well have the Danish instead.

Also, with the proliferation of coffee shops there is a big temptation to make coffee your midmorning or late afternoon snack. The caffeine in coffee does pick you up—temporarily. But it does not provide you with any real energy (because it doesn't provide calories to burn), and can actually drive up hunger, causing your existing energy levels to drop even further.

• **Follow the one-hour rule:** You eat to recover and to keep energy levels up, and there is no more crucial moment for food than following a hard workout, like a long run, tempo run, hill run, or track workout. In fact, studies have shown that a key time to eat following these workouts (when you will be depleted of carbs and your muscles will be sore) is within an hour of finishing. This "one-hour window" is when your body will be hungering for those lost carbs and is more likely to replace them. It's also a good time to begin the recovery process for those damaged muscle tissues. So you want to eat something less than sixty minutes after your hard workout has ended to facilitate both of these processes. Energy bars can come in handy at this time because you can take them to your workout venue, then eat them soon after. Also, some protein, in addition to carbohydrates, has been shown to be beneficial because protein helps in muscle recovery. So look for an energy bar with protein—or you can pack something at the deli like half a tuna-fish sandwich on whole wheat bread.

• **See red on your plate:** During the pasta boom of the 1990s, red meat got a bad name among runners. Since then, however, steaks and burgers have been making a comeback. And for good reason: Probably no food has the ability to help your recover and bounce back from a hard workout (or withstand the constant stress of a four-month training program, like this one) than red meat. Packed with protein and iron and all sorts of good stuff, red meat can be your food secret in your quest for a PR.

If you are a vegetarian, however, don't disrupt your diet (because to force anything radically new during training will only add stress). But if you are a carnivore and have simply been avoiding red meat, then you should consider adding it on occasion throughout the training program. Choose lean cuts of meat and don't have cheese and onion rings with your burger. At the most, eat red meat twice a week because it takes a while to digest, and this could cause stomach distress during a workout.

• **Eat out wisely:** Runners like to eat out. There is no denying it. This should not become a problem as long as the keys to eating out wisely are observed—make healthy choices and watch portion size. If you can substitute a baked potato for French fries (making a healthy choice) and order just two pancakes for breakfast not four (watching portion size), there is no reason why you cannot eat out a several times a week—if you so desire and your budget allows. Besides, eating out has a way of breaking up the training week the way nothing else quite can.

Yet there is danger in eating out, an aspect to eating out that is often overlooked. And that is the reward meal, a splurge for something unhealthy and filling as a prize for all the hard running you have been doing. The reward meal has the potential to stop you cold if it becomes habit. Fortunately, there is a safe way to deal with this phenomenon. The first thing you need to do is eat a healthy snack soon after completing your hard workout. This will stop the hunger pangs and cravings and temporarily cut off that connection between running and food. The second thing you need to do is to eat your postrace meal soon afterward. This does two things: It makes sure you are getting fuel when your body needs it the most (postworkout). It also gets you sitting down for your meal while your snack is still working to keep those hunger pangs down. This is especially important when you go out for that meal and the temptation—because you have done such a hard workout and are so hungry—will be to order half the menu, with cheese. That is, when you are tempted to have a reward meal.

Yet, having said all that, the concept of a reward meal is not such a bad thing and one such meal every other week or so can actually help reduce stress during the training process, leaving you fresher for your running than you might have been before. The trick is to know when to eat it. You want to eat it when the connection between running and food is at its lowest, and that would be on an easy day or on your day off. Having a reward meal on one of these days makes sure you are eating your reward meal when hunger is relatively low (compared to a day when you have run a hard workout). This will make portion size easier to manage, so that you can safely order the deep-dish pizza, knowing that you are going for a small with one topping (with a nice salad, perhaps) and not the large with everything.

The Weekend Naps

Here is what you need to know about elite runners when they are training for high-level competition:

They run a lot.

They eat a lot.

And they sleep a lot.

Not just eight hours a night (though they probably average more than eight) but plenty of nap time during the day between their morning runs and evening runs. It is the only way they can train at such a high level month after month after month.

Now, most of you cannot negotiate a weekday siesta—because of work or school or both—but there are two days when you could possibly squeeze them in: Saturday and Sunday. Napping on these days is a great way to recover from the training week behind you and to prepare for the training week ahead. You might also make this discovery—your weekend naps help you sleep more soundly on Saturday and Sunday (because you are not over-tired at bedtime), adding to the effectiveness of sleep at this crucial moment in your training week.

Therefore, try to find an hour or so in a quiet room on these days. Lie down, cover up, close your eyes, and nap. Once you get into the habit your body will begin to anticipate these naps and you should fall asleep more quickly.

Note: Sleep plays a vital role in your quest for a PR. If you can't find the time to nap and feel you need extra sleep, try going to bed earlier (by a half hour or an hour) a couple times a week, particularly the night before a hard workout.

CHAPTER 6

The PR Schedules

This chapter is where we get down to it. I have taken the four most popular race distances (the 5K, 10K, half marathon, and marathon) and laid out four training programs for each, focusing on the most popular PR time goals for each. For example, the four training programs for the 5K are 22:30, 25:00, 27:30, and 30:00. The four training programs for the half marathon are 1:50, 2:00, 2:10, and 2:20.

These training schedules are your road map to a particular PR. Once you decide on a particular PR goal and schedule, you should try to stick as closely as possible to the schedule, writing down your progress in the training log section of this book.

Note: The Road Work and Strength Work schedule for each distance is a general one, and should be applied to each training schedule, no matter what your time goal. Then pick up the specific time goal training schedule for your Track Work phase. For instance, complete the eight weeks of Road Work and three weeks of Strength Work for a 5K, then plug into the 25-minute training program for your Track Work.

To begin your PR training regimen, figure out what race distance you want to tackle this season. Decide on your time goal. Count back seventeen weeks (four months, plus one prerace week) from your designated race. Then begin your day-by-day training program to be able to run a PR on race day. Write your goals here.

Your race distance:

Your time goal:

If you're running a 5K, turn to page 59.

If you're running a 10K, turn to page 70.

If you're running a half marathon, turn to page 81.

If you're running a marathon, turn to page 92.

THE 5K

Road Work and Strength Work for all 5K schedules

Week 1

Road Work

MONDAY:	4 miles easy
TUESDAY:	3 miles easy
WEDNESDAY:	5 miles easy
THURSDAY:	3 miles easy or off
FRIDAY:	3 miles easy
SATURDAY:	5 miles easy
SUNDAY:	off

Week 2

Road Work

MONDAY:	4 miles easy
TUESDAY:	3 miles easy
WEDNESDAY:	5 miles easy
THURSDAY:	3 miles easy or off
FRIDAY:	3 miles easy
SATURDAY:	6 miles easy
SUNDAY:	off

Week 3

Road Work

MONDAY:	5 miles easy
TUESDAY:	4 miles easy
WEDNESDAY:	5 miles easy
THURSDAY:	3 miles easy or off
FRIDAY:	4 miles easy
SATURDAY:	6 miles easy
SUNDAY:	off

Week 4

Road Work

MONDAY:	5 miles easy
TUESDAY:	4 miles easy; 4 striders
WEDNESDAY:	5 miles easy
THURSDAY:	3 miles easy or off
FRIDAY:	4 miles easy; 4 striders
SATURDAY:	6 miles easy
SUNDAY:	off

The 5K

Road Work

Week 5		
MONDAY:	5 miles easy
TUESDAY:	4 miles easy; 4 striders
WEDNESDAY:	5 miles easy
THURSDAY:	3 miles easy or off
FRIDAY:	4 miles easy; 4 striders
SATURDAY:	6 miles easy
SUNDAY:	off

Road Work

Week 6		
MONDAY:	5 miles easy
TUESDAY:	4 miles easy; 6 striders
WEDNESDAY:	6 miles easy
THURSDAY:	3 miles easy or off
FRIDAY:	4 miles easy; 6 striders
SATURDAY:	7 miles easy
SUNDAY:	off

Road Work

Week 7		
MONDAY:	5 miles easy
TUESDAY:	4 miles easy; 6 striders
WEDNESDAY:	6 miles easy
THURSDAY:	3 miles easy or off
FRIDAY:	4 miles easy; 6 striders
SATURDAY:	8 miles easy
SUNDAY:	off

Road Work

Week 8		
MONDAY:	5 miles easy
TUESDAY:	4 miles easy; 6 striders
WEDNESDAY:	7 miles easy
THURSDAY:	3 miles easy or off
FRIDAY:	4 miles easy; 6 striders
SATURDAY:	8 miles easy
SUNDAY:	off

The 5K

Strength Work

Week 9		
	MONDAY:	5 miles easy
	TUESDAY:	1 mile warm-up; 4 x hill; 1 mile cooldown
	WEDNESDAY:	3 miles easy or off
	THURSDAY:	1 mile warm-up; 20-minute tempo run; 1 mile cooldown
	FRIDAY:	3 miles easy or off
	SATURDAY:	8 miles easy
	SUNDAY:	off

Strength Work

Week 10		
	MONDAY:	5 miles easy
	TUESDAY:	1 mile warm-up; 6 x hill; 1 mile cooldown
	WEDNESDAY:	3 miles easy or off
	THURSDAY:	1 mile warm-up; 20-minute tempo run; 1 mile cooldown
	FRIDAY:	3 miles easy or off
	SATURDAY:	8 miles easy
	SUNDAY:	off

Strength Work

Week 11		
	MONDAY:	5 miles easy
	TUESDAY:	1 mile warm-up; 8 x hill; 1 mile cooldown
	WEDNESDAY:	3 miles easy or off
	THURSDAY:	1 mile warm-up; 20-minute tempo run; 1 mile cooldown
	FRIDAY:	3 miles easy or off
	SATURDAY:	8 miles easy
	SUNDAY:	off

The 5K

THE 22:30 5K

To run a 5K in 22 minutes and 30 seconds, you need to average 7 minutes and 14 seconds per mile.

Track Work

Week 12		
MONDAY:	5 miles easy
TUESDAY:	1 mile warm-up, plus 4 striders; 6 x 400 at 1:40–1:45; 1 mile cooldown
WEDNESDAY:	3 miles easy or off
THURSDAY:	1 mile warm-up, plus 4 striders; 3 × 800 at 3:38; 1 mile cooldown
FRIDAY:	3 miles easy or off
SATURDAY:	8 miles easy
SUNDAY:	off

Track Work

Week 13		
MONDAY:	5 miles easy
TUESDAY:	1 mile warm-up, plus 4 striders; 8 x 400 at 1:40–1:45; 1 mile cooldown
WEDNESDAY:	3 miles easy or off
THURSDAY:	1 mile warm-up, plus 4 striders; 4 x 800 at 3:38; 1 mile cooldown
FRIDAY:	3 miles easy or off
SATURDAY:	8 miles easy
SUNDAY:	off

Track Work

Week 14		
MONDAY:	5 miles easy
TUESDAY:	1 mile warm-up, plus 4 striders; 10 x 400 at 1:40–1:45; 1 mile cooldown
WEDNESDAY:	3 miles easy or off
THURSDAY:	1 mile warm-up, plus 4 striders; 2 x 1 mile at 7:14; 1 mile cooldown
FRIDAY:	3 miles easy or off
SATURDAY:	8 miles easy
SUNDAY:	off

The 5K

Week 15

Track Work

MONDAY:	5 miles easy
TUESDAY:	1 mile warm-up, plus 4 striders; 12 x 400 at 1:40–1:45; 1 mile cooldown
WEDNESDAY:	3 miles easy or off
THURSDAY:	1 mile warm-up, plus 4 striders; 3 x 1 mile at 7:14; 1 mile cooldown
FRIDAY:	3 miles easy or off
SATURDAY:	8 miles easy
SUNDAY:	off

Week 16

Track Work

MONDAY:	5 miles easy
TUESDAY:	1 mile warm-up, plus 4 striders; 1 mile in 7:14, 3/4 mile in 5:23, 800 in 3:30, 400 in 1:40; 1 mile cooldown
WEDNESDAY:	3 miles easy or off
THURSDAY:	1 mile warm-up, plus 4 striders; 3 x 1 mile in 7:14; 1 mile cooldown
FRIDAY:	3 miles easy or off
SATURDAY:	8 miles easy
SUNDAY:	off

Race Week

Track Work

MONDAY:	4 miles easy
TUESDAY:	1 mile warm-up, plus 4 striders; 6 x 400 in 1:49; 1 mile cooldown
WEDNESDAY:	off
THURSDAY:	off
FRIDAY:	2 miles easy
SATURDAY:	RACE
SUNDAY:	Rest, recover, and celebrate

The 5K

THE 25:00 5K

To run a 5K in 25 minutes you need to average 8 minutes and 3 seconds per mile.

Track Work

Week 12		
	MONDAY:	5 miles easy
	TUESDAY:	1 mile warm-up, plus 4 striders; 6 x 400 at 1:50–1:55; 1 mile cooldown
	WEDNESDAY:	3 miles easy or off
	THURSDAY:	1 mile warm-up, plus 4 striders; 3 x 800 at 4:01; 1 mile cooldown
	FRIDAY:	3 miles easy or off
	SATURDAY:	8 miles easy
	SUNDAY:	off

Track Work

Week 13		
	MONDAY:	5 miles easy
	TUESDAY:	1 mile warm-up, plus 4 striders; 8 x 400 at 1:50–1:55; 1 mile cooldown
	WEDNESDAY:	3 miles easy or off
	THURSDAY:	1 mile warm-up, plus 4 striders; 4 x 800 at 4:01; 1 mile cooldown
	FRIDAY:	3 miles easy or off
	SATURDAY:	8 miles easy
	SUNDAY:	off

Track Work

Week 14		
	MONDAY:	5 miles easy
	TUESDAY:	1 mile warm-up, plus 4 striders; 10 x 400 at 1:50–1:55; 1 mile cooldown
	WEDNESDAY:	3 miles easy or off
	THURSDAY:	1 mile warm-up, plus 4 striders; 2 x 1 mile at 8:03; 1 mile cooldown
	FRIDAY:	3 miles easy or off
	SATURDAY:	8 miles easy
	SUNDAY:	off

The 5K

Track Work

Week 15		
MONDAY:	5 miles easy
TUESDAY:	1 mile warm-up, plus 4 striders; 12 × 400 at 1:50–1:55; 1 mile cooldown
WEDNESDAY:	3 miles easy or off
THURSDAY:	1 mile warm-up, plus 4 striders; 3 × 1 mile at 8:03; 1 mile cooldown
FRIDAY:	3 miles easy or off
SATURDAY:	8 miles easy
SUNDAY:	off

Track Work

Week 16		
MONDAY:	5 miles easy
TUESDAY:	1 mile warm-up, plus 4 striders; 1 mile in 8:03, 3/4 in 5:57; 800 in 3:53; 400 in 1:50; 1 mile cooldown
WEDNESDAY:	3 miles easy or off
THURSDAY:	1 mile warm-up, plus 4 striders; 3 x 1 mile in 8:03; 1 mile cooldown
FRIDAY:	3 miles easy or off
SATURDAY:	8 miles easy
SUNDAY:	off

Track Work

Race Week		
MONDAY:	4 miles easy
TUESDAY:	1 mile warm-up, plus 4 striders; 6 × 400 in 2:00; 1 mile cooldown
WEDNESDAY:	off
THURSDAY:	off
FRIDAY:	2 miles
SATURDAY:	RACE
SUNDAY:	Rest, recover, and celebrate

The 5K

THE 27:30 5K

To run a 5K in 27 minutes and 30 seconds you need to average 8 minutes and 51 seconds per mile.

Track Work

Week 12		
	MONDAY:	5 miles easy
	TUESDAY:	1 mile warm-up, plus 4 striders; 6 x 400 in 2:02–2:07; 1 mile cooldown
	WEDNESDAY:	3 miles easy or off
	THURSDAY:	1 mile warm-up, plus 4 striders; 3 x 800 in 4:25; 1 mile cooldown
	FRIDAY:	3 miles easy or off
	SATURDAY:	8 miles easy
	SUNDAY:	off

Track Work

Week 13		
	MONDAY:	5 miles easy
	TUESDAY:	1 mile warm-up, plus 4 striders; 8 x 400 in 2:02–2:07; 1 mile cooldown
	WEDNESDAY:	3 miles easy or off
	THURSDAY:	1 mile warm-up, plus 4 striders; 4 x 800 in 4:25; 1 mile cooldown
	FRIDAY:	3 miles easy or off
	SATURDAY:	8 miles easy
	SUNDAY:	off

Track Work

Week 14		
	MONDAY:	5 miles easy
	TUESDAY:	1 mile warm-up, plus 4 striders; 10 x 400 in 2:02–2:07; 1 mile cooldown
	WEDNESDAY:	3 miles easy or off
	THURSDAY:	1 mile warm-up, plus 4 striders; 2 x 1 mile in 8:51; 1 mile cooldown
	FRIDAY:	3 miles easy or off
	SATURDAY:	8 miles easy
	SUNDAY:	off

The 5K

Track Work

MONDAY:	5 miles easy
TUESDAY:	1 mile warm-up, plus 4 striders; 12 x 400 in 2:02–2:07; 1 mile cooldown
WEDNESDAY:	3 miles easy or off
THURSDAY:	1 mile warm-up, plus 4 striders; 3 x 1 mile in 8:51: 1 mile cooldown
FRIDAY:	3 miles easy or off
SATURDAY:	8 miles easy
SUNDAY:	off

Week 15

Track Work

MONDAY:	5 miles easy
TUESDAY:	1 mile warm-up, plus 4 striders; 1 mile in 8:51, I mile in 6:33, 800 in 4:18, 400 in 2:02; 1 mile cooldown
WEDNESDAY:	3 miles easy or off
THURSDAY:	1 mile warm-up, plus 4 striders; 3 x 1 mile in 8:51; 1 mile cooldown
FRIDAY:	3 miles easy or off
SATURDAY:	8 miles easy
SUNDAY:	off

Week 16

Track Work

MONDAY:	4 miles easy
TUESDAY:	1 mile warm-up, plus 4 striders; 6 x 400 in 2:12; 1 mile cooldown
WEDNESDAY:	off
THURSDAY:	off
FRIDAY:	2 miles easy
SATURDAY:	RACE
SUNDAY:	Rest, recover, and celebrate

Race Week

The 5K

THE 30:00 5K

To run a 5K in 30 minutes you need to average 9 minutes and 39 seconds per mile.

Track Work

Week 12		
	MONDAY:	5 miles easy
	TUESDAY:	1 mile warm-up, plus 4 striders; 6 × 400 at 2:15–2:20; 1 mile cooldown
	WEDNESDAY:	3 miles easy or off
	THURSDAY:	1 mile warm-up, plus 4 striders; 3 × 800 at 4:49; 1 mile cooldown
	FRIDAY:	3 miles easy or off
	SATURDAY:	8 miles easy
	SUNDAY:	off

Track Work

Week 13		
	MONDAY:	5 miles easy
	TUESDAY:	1 mile warm-up, plus 4 striders; 8 × 400 at 2:15–2:20; 1 mile cooldown
	WEDNESDAY:	3 miles easy or off
	THURSDAY:	1 mile warm-up, plus 4 striders; 4 × 800 at 4:49; 1 mile cooldown
	FRIDAY:	3 miles easy or off
	SATURDAY:	8 miles easy
	SUNDAY:	off

Track Work

Week 14		
	MONDAY:	5 miles easy
	TUESDAY:	1 mile warm-up, plus 4 striders; 10 × 400 at 2:15–2:20; 1 mile cooldown
	WEDNESDAY:	3 miles easy or off
	THURSDAY:	1 mile warm-up, plus 4 striders; 2 × 1 mile at 9:39; 1 mile cooldown
	FRIDAY:	3 miles easy or off
	SATURDAY:	8 miles easy
	SUNDAY:	off

The 5K

Week 15

Track Work

MONDAY:	5 miles easy
TUESDAY:	1 mile warm-up, plus 4 striders; 12 × 400 at 2:15–2:20; 1 mile cooldown
WEDNESDAY:	3 miles easy or off
THURSDAY:	1 mile warm-up, plus 4 striders; 3 × 1 mile at 9:39; 1 mile cooldown
FRIDAY:	3 miles easy or off
SATURDAY:	8 miles easy
SUNDAY:	off

Week 16

Track Work

MONDAY:	5 miles easy
TUESDAY:	1 mile warm-up, plus 4 striders; 1 mile in 9:39, ¾ in 7:12, 800 in 4:43, 400 in 2:15; 1 mile cooldown
WEDNESDAY:	3 miles easy or off
THURSDAY:	1 mile warm-up, plus 4 striders; 3 × 1 mile in 9:39; 1 mile cooldown
FRIDAY:	3 miles easy or off
SATURDAY:	8 miles easy
SUNDAY:	off

Race Week

Track Work

MONDAY:	4 miles easy
TUESDAY:	1 mile warm-up, plus 4 striders; 6 × 400 in 2:25; 1 mile cooldown
WEDNESDAY:	off
THURSDAY:	off
FRIDAY:	2 miles
SATURDAY:	RACE
SUNDAY:	Rest, recover, and celebrate

THE 10K

Road Work and Strength Work for all 10K schedules

Road Work

MONDAY:	5 miles easy
TUESDAY:	4 miles easy
WEDNESDAY:	5 miles easy
THURSDAY:	3 miles easy or off
FRIDAY:	4 miles easy
SATURDAY:	6 miles easy
SUNDAY:	off

Road Work

Week 2

MONDAY:	5 miles easy
TUESDAY:	4 miles easy
WEDNESDAY:	5 miles easy
THURSDAY:	3 miles easy or off
FRIDAY:	4 miles easy
SATURDAY:	7 miles easy
SUNDAY:	off

Road Work

Week 3

MONDAY:	6 miles easy
TUESDAY:	5 miles easy
WEDNESDAY:	6 miles easy
THURSDAY:	3 miles easy or off
FRIDAY:	5 miles easy
SATURDAY:	7 miles easy
SUNDAY:	off

Road Work

Week 4

MONDAY:	6 miles easy
TUESDAY:	5 miles easy; 4 striders
WEDNESDAY:	6 miles easy
THURSDAY:	3 miles easy or off
FRIDAY:	5 miles easy; 4 striders
SATURDAY:	8 miles easy
SUNDAY:	off

The 10K

Road Work

MONDAY:	6 miles easy
TUESDAY:	5 miles easy; 4 striders
WEDNESDAY:	6 miles easy
THURSDAY:	off
FRIDAY:	5 miles easy; 4 striders
SATURDAY:	8 miles easy
SUNDAY:	off

Road Work

Week 6

MONDAY:	6 miles easy
TUESDAY:	5 miles easy; 6 striders
WEDNESDAY:	7 miles easy
THURSDAY:	off
FRIDAY:	5 miles easy; 6 striders
SATURDAY:	9 miles easy
SUNDAY:	off

Road Work

Week 7

MONDAY:	6 miles easy
TUESDAY:	5 miles easy; 6 striders
WEDNESDAY:	8 miles easy
THURSDAY:	off
FRIDAY:	5 miles easy; 6 striders
SATURDAY:	10 miles easy
SUNDAY:	off

Road Work

Week 8

MONDAY:	6 miles easy
TUESDAY:	5 miles easy; 6 striders
WEDNESDAY:	8 miles easy
THURSDAY:	off
FRIDAY:	5 miles easy; 6 striders
SATURDAY:	10 miles easy
SUNDAY:	off

The 10K

Strength Work

<table>
<tr><td rowspan="7">Week 9</td><td>MONDAY:</td><td>6 miles easy</td></tr>
<tr><td>TUESDAY:</td><td>2 mile warm-up; 6 × hill; 2 mile cooldown</td></tr>
<tr><td>WEDNESDAY:</td><td>4 miles easy or off</td></tr>
<tr><td>THURSDAY:</td><td>2 mile warm-up; 20-minute tempo run; 2 mile cooldown</td></tr>
<tr><td>FRIDAY:</td><td>4 miles easy or off</td></tr>
<tr><td>SATURDAY:</td><td>10 miles easy</td></tr>
<tr><td>SUNDAY:</td><td>off</td></tr>
</table>

Strength Work

<table>
<tr><td rowspan="7">Week 10</td><td>MONDAY:</td><td>6 miles easy</td></tr>
<tr><td>TUESDAY:</td><td>2 mile warm-up; 8 × hill; 2 mile cooldown</td></tr>
<tr><td>WEDNESDAY:</td><td>4 miles easy or off</td></tr>
<tr><td>THURSDAY:</td><td>2 mile warm-up; 20-minute tempo run; 2 mile cooldown</td></tr>
<tr><td>FRIDAY:</td><td>4 miles easy or off</td></tr>
<tr><td>SATURDAY:</td><td>10 miles easy</td></tr>
<tr><td>SUNDAY:</td><td>off</td></tr>
</table>

Strength Work

<table>
<tr><td rowspan="7">Week 11</td><td>MONDAY:</td><td>6 miles easy</td></tr>
<tr><td>TUESDAY:</td><td>2 mile warm-up; 10 x hill; 2 mile cooldown</td></tr>
<tr><td>WEDNESDAY:</td><td>4 miles easy or off</td></tr>
<tr><td>THURSDAY:</td><td>2 mile warm-up; 20-minute tempo run; 2 mile cooldown</td></tr>
<tr><td>FRIDAY:</td><td>4 miles easy or off</td></tr>
<tr><td>SATURDAY:</td><td>10 miles easy</td></tr>
<tr><td>SUNDAY:</td><td>off</td></tr>
</table>

The 10K

THE 45:00 10K

To run a 10K in 45 minutes you need to average 7 minutes and 14 seconds per mile.

Week 12

Track Work

MONDAY:	6 miles easy
TUESDAY:	2 mile warm-up, plus 4 striders; 8 × 400 in 1:38–1:43; 2 mile cooldown
WEDNESDAY:	4 miles easy or off
THURSDAY:	2 mile warm-up, plus 4 striders; 4 × 800 in 3:37; 2 mile cooldown
FRIDAY:	4 miles easy or off
SATURDAY:	10 miles easy
SUNDAY:	off

Week 13

Track Work

MONDAY:	6 miles easy
TUESDAY:	2 mile warm-up, plus 4 striders; 10 × 400 in 1:38–1:42; 2 mile cooldown
WEDNESDAY:	4 miles easy or off
THURSDAY:	2 mile warm-up, plus 4 striders; 5 × 800 in 3:37; 2 mile cooldown
FRIDAY:	4 miles easy or off
SATURDAY:	10 miles easy
SUNDAY:	off

Week 14

Track Work

MONDAY:	6 miles easy
TUESDAY:	2 mile warm-up, plus 4 striders; 12 × 400 in 1:38–1:42; 2 mile cooldown
WEDNESDAY:	4 miles easy or off
THURSDAY:	2 mile warm-up, plus 4 striders; 3 × 1 mile in 7:14; 2 mile cooldown
FRIDAY:	4 miles easy or off
SATURDAY:	10 miles easy
SUNDAY:	off

The 10K

Track Work

Week 15		
	MONDAY:	6 miles easy
	TUESDAY:	2 mile warm-up, plus 4 striders; 12 × 400 in 1:38–1:42; 2 mile cooldown
	WEDNESDAY:	4 miles easy or off
	THURSDAY:	2 mile warm-up, plus 4 striders; 4 × 1 mile in 7:14; 2 mile cooldown
	FRIDAY:	4 miles easy or off
	SATURDAY:	10 miles easy
	SUNDAY:	off

Track Work

Week 16		
	MONDAY:	6 miles easy
	TUESDAY:	2 mile warm-up, plus 4 striders; 2 miles at 7:14 pace, 1 mile at 7:05, 800 at 3:30, 400 at 1:38; 2 mile cooldown
	WEDNESDAY:	4 miles easy or off
	THURSDAY:	2 mile warm-up, plus 4 striders; 4 × 1 mile in 7:14; 2 mile cooldown
	FRIDAY:	4 miles easy or off
	SATURDAY:	8 miles easy
	SUNDAY:	off

Track Work

Race Week		
	MONDAY:	5 miles easy
	TUESDAY:	2 mile warm-up, plus 4 striders; 8 × 400 in 1:48; 2 mile cooldown
	WEDNESDAY:	off
	THURSDAY:	off
	FRIDAY:	3 miles easy
	SATURDAY:	RACE
	SUNDAY:	Rest, recover, and celebrate

The 10K

THE 50:00 10K

To run a 10K in 50 minutes you need to average 8 minutes and 3 seconds per mile.

Track Work

Week 12		
	MONDAY:	6 miles easy
	TUESDAY:	2 mile warm-up, plus 4 striders; 8 × 400 at 1:50–1:55; 2 mile cooldown
	WEDNESDAY:	4 miles easy or off
	THURSDAY:	2 mile warm-up, plus 4 striders; 4 × 800 in 4:01; 2 mile cooldown
	FRIDAY:	4 miles easy or off
	SATURDAY:	10 miles easy
	SUNDAY:	off

Track Work

Week 13		
	MONDAY:	6 miles easy
	TUESDAY:	2 mile warm-up, plus 4 striders; 10 × 400 at 1:50–1:55; 2 mile cooldown
	WEDNESDAY:	4 miles easy or off
	THURSDAY:	2 mile warm-up, plus 4 striders; 5 × 800 in 4:01; 2 mile cooldown
	FRIDAY:	4 miles easy
	SATURDAY:	10 miles easy
	SUNDAY:	off

Track Work

Week 14		
	MONDAY:	6 miles easy
	TUESDAY:	2 mile warm-up, plus 4 striders; 12 × 400 at 1:50–1:55; 2 mile cooldown
	WEDNESDAY:	4 miles easy or off
	THURSDAY:	2 mile warm-up, plus 4 striders; 3 × 1 mile at 8:03; 2 mile cooldown
	FRIDAY:	4 miles easy or off
	SATURDAY:	10 miles easy
	SUNDAY:	off

Track Work

Week 15		
	MONDAY:	6 miles easy
	TUESDAY:	2 mile warm-up, plus 4 striders; 12 × 400 at 1:50–1:55; 2 mile cooldown
	WEDNESDAY:	4 miles easy or off
	THURSDAY:	2 mile warm-up, plus 4 striders; 4 × 1 mile at 8:03; 2 mile cooldown
	FRIDAY:	4 miles easy or off
	SATURDAY:	10 miles easy
	SUNDAY:	off

Track Work

Week 16		
	MONDAY:	6 miles easy
	TUESDAY:	2 mile warm-up, plus 4 striders; 2 miles in 16:06, 1 mile in 7:58, 800 in 3:53, 400 in 1:50; 2 mile cooldown
	WEDNESDAY:	4 miles easy or off
	THURSDAY:	2 mile warm-up, plus 4 striders; 4 × 1 mile at 8:03; 2 mile cooldown
	FRIDAY:	4 miles easy or off
	SATURDAY:	8 miles easy
	SUNDAY:	off

Track Work

Race Week		
	MONDAY:	5 miles easy
	TUESDAY:	2 mile warm-up, plus 4 striders; 8 × 400 in 2:00; 2 mile cooldown
	WEDNESDAY:	off
	THURSDAY:	off
	FRIDAY:	3 miles easy
	SATURDAY:	RACE
	SUNDAY:	Rest, recover, and celebrate

The 10K

THE 55:00 10K

To run a 10K in 55 minutes you need to average 8 minutes and 51 seconds per mile.

Week 12

Track Work

MONDAY:	6 miles easy
TUESDAY:	2 mile warm-up, plus 4 striders; 8 × 400 at 2:02–2:07; 2 mile cooldown
WEDNESDAY:	4 miles easy or off
THURSDAY:	2 mile warm-up, plus 4 striders; 4 × 800 in 4:25; 2 mile cooldown
FRIDAY:	4 miles easy or off
SATURDAY:	10 miles easy
SUNDAY:	off

Week 13

Track Work

MONDAY:	6 miles easy
TUESDAY:	2 mile warm-up, plus 4 striders; 10 × 400 at 2:02–2:07; 2 mile cooldown
WEDNESDAY:	4 miles easy or off
THURSDAY:	2 mile warm-up, plus 4 striders; 5 × 800 in 4:25; 2 mile cooldown
FRIDAY:	4 miles easy or off
SATURDAY:	10 miles easy
SUNDAY:	off

Week 14

Track Work

MONDAY:	6 miles easy
TUESDAY:	2 mile warm-up, plus 4 striders; 12 × 400 at 2:02–2:07; 2 mile cooldown
WEDNESDAY:	4 miles easy or off
THURSDAY:	2 mile warm-up, plus 4 striders; 3 × 1 mile in 8:51; 2 mile cooldown
FRIDAY:	4 miles easy or off
SATURDAY:	10 miles easy
SUNDAY:	off

The 10K

Track Work

Week 15		
MONDAY:	6 miles easy
TUESDAY:	2 mile warm-up, plus 4 striders; 12 × 400 at 2:02–2:07; 2 mile cooldown
WEDNESDAY:	4 miles easy or off
THURSDAY:	2 mile warm-up, plus 4 striders; 4 × 1 mile in 8:51; 2 mile cooldown
FRIDAY:	4 miles easy or off
SATURDAY:	10 miles easy
SUNDAY:	off

Track Work

Week 16		
MONDAY:	6 miles easy
TUESDAY:	2 mile warm-up, plus 4 striders; 2 miles in 17:42, 1 mile in 8:46, 800 in 4:17, 400 in 2:02; 2 mile cooldown
WEDNESDAY:	4 miles easy or off
THURSDAY:	2 mile warm-up, plus 4 striders; 4 × 1 mile in 8:51; 2 mile cooldown
FRIDAY:	4 miles easy or off
SATURDAY:	8 miles easy
SUNDAY:	off

Track Work

Race Week		
MONDAY:	5 miles easy
TUESDAY:	2 mile warm-up, plus 4 striders; 8 × 400 in 2:12; 2 mile cooldown
WEDNESDAY:	off
THURSDAY:	off
FRIDAY:	3 miles easy
SATURDAY:	RACE
SUNDAY:	Rest, recover, and celebrate

The 10K

THE 60:00 10K

To run a 10K in 60 minutes you need to average 9 minutes and 39 seconds per mile.

Track Work

Week 12		
MONDAY:	6 miles easy
TUESDAY:	2 mile warm-up, plus 4 striders; 8 × 400 at 2:14–2:19; 2 mile cooldown
WEDNESDAY:	4 miles easy or off
THURSDAY:	2 mile warm-up, plus 4 striders; 4 × 800 at 4:49; 2 mile cooldown
FRIDAY:	4 miles easy or off
SATURDAY:	10 miles easy
SUNDAY:	off

Track Work

Week 13		
MONDAY:	6 miles easy
TUESDAY:	2 mile warm-up, plus 4 striders; 10 × 400 at 2:14–2:19; 2 mile cooldown
WEDNESDAY:	4 miles easy or off
THURSDAY:	2 mile warm-up, plus 4 striders; 5 × 800 at 4:49; 2 mile cooldown
FRIDAY:	4 miles easy or off
SATURDAY:	10 miles easy
SUNDAY:	off

Track Work

Week 14		
MONDAY:	6 miles easy
TUESDAY:	2 mile warm-up, plus 4 striders; 12 × 400 at 2:14–2:19; 2 mile cooldown
WEDNESDAY:	4 miles easy or off
THURSDAY:	2 mile warm-up, plus 4 striders; 3 × 1 mile at 9:39; 2 mile cooldown
FRIDAY:	4 miles easy or off
SATURDAY:	10 miles easy
SUNDAY:	off

The 10K

Track Work

Week 15		
	MONDAY:	6 miles easy
	TUESDAY:	2 mile warm-up, plus 4 striders; 12 × 400 at 2:14–2:19; 2 mile cooldown
	WEDNESDAY:	4 miles easy or off
	THURSDAY:	2 mile warm-up, plus 4 striders; 4 × 1 mile at 9:39; 2 mile cooldown
	FRIDAY:	4 miles easy or off
	SATURDAY:	10 miles easy

Track Work

Week 16		
	MONDAY:	6 miles easy
	TUESDAY:	2 mile warm-up, plus 4 striders; 2 miles in 19:18, 1 mile in 9:34, 800 in 4:42, 400 in 2:14; 2 mile cooldown
	WEDNESDAY:	4 miles easy or off
	THURSDAY:	2 mile warm-up, plus 4 striders; 4 × 1 mile in 9:39; 2 mile cooldown
	FRIDAY:	4 miles easy or off
	SATURDAY:	8 miles easy
	SUNDAY:	off

Track Work

Race Week		
	MONDAY:	5 miles easy
	TUESDAY:	2 mile warm-up, plus 4 striders; 8 × 400 in 2:24; 2 mile cooldown
	WEDNESDAY:	off
	THURSDAY:	off
	FRIDAY:	3 miles easy
	SATURDAY:	RACE
	SUNDAY:	Rest, recover, and celebrate

The 10K

THE HALF MARATHON
Road Work and Strength Work for all half marathon schedules

Week 1

Road Work

MONDAY:	6 miles easy
TUESDAY:	5 miles easy
WEDNESDAY:	6 miles easy
THURSDAY:	4 miles easy or off
FRIDAY:	4 miles easy
SATURDAY:	8 miles easy
SUNDAY:	off

Week 2

Road Work

MONDAY:	6 miles easy
TUESDAY:	5 miles easy
WEDNESDAY:	7 miles easy
THURSDAY:	4 miles easy or off
FRIDAY:	4 miles easy
SATURDAY:	9 miles easy
SUNDAY:	off

Week 3

Road Work

MONDAY:	7 miles easy
TUESDAY:	6 miles easy
WEDNESDAY:	7 miles easy
THURSDAY:	4 miles easy or off
FRIDAY:	5 miles easy
SATURDAY:	9 miles easy
SUNDAY:	off

Week 4

Road Work

MONDAY:	7 miles easy
TUESDAY:	6 miles easy; 6 striders
WEDNESDAY:	8 miles easy
THURSDAY:	4 miles easy or off
FRIDAY:	5 miles easy; 6 striders
SATURDAY:	10 miles easy
SUNDAY:	off

The Half Marathon

The Half Marathon

Road Work

Week 5		
	MONDAY:	7 miles easy
	TUESDAY:	6 miles easy; 6 striders
	WEDNESDAY:	8 miles easy
	THURSDAY:	4 miles easy or off
	FRIDAY:	5 miles easy; 6 striders
	SATURDAY:	10 miles easy
	SUNDAY:	off

Road Work

Week 6		
	MONDAY:	7 miles easy
	TUESDAY:	6 miles easy; 8 striders
	WEDNESDAY:	8 miles easy
	THURSDAY:	4 miles easy or off
	FRIDAY:	5 miles easy; 8 striders
	SATURDAY:	12 miles easy
	SUNDAY:	off

Road Work

Week 7		
	MONDAY:	7 miles easy
	TUESDAY:	6 miles easy; 8 striders
	WEDNESDAY:	8 miles easy
	THURSDAY:	4 miles easy or off
	FRIDAY:	5 miles easy; 8 striders
	SATURDAY:	14 miles easy
	SUNDAY:	off

Road Work

Week 8		
	MONDAY:	7 miles easy
	TUESDAY:	6 miles easy; 8 striders
	WEDNESDAY:	8 miles easy
	THURSDAY:	4 miles easy or off
	FRIDAY:	5 miles easy; 8 striders
	SATURDAY:	16 miles easy
	SUNDAY:	off

Strength Work

	Week 9
MONDAY:	7 miles easy
TUESDAY:	2 mile warm-up; 8 × hill; 2 mile cooldown
WEDNESDAY:	4 miles easy or off
THURSDAY:	2 mile warm-up; 40-minute tempo run; 2 mile cooldown
FRIDAY:	4 miles easy or off
SATURDAY:	12 miles easy
SUNDAY:	off

Strength Work

	Week 10
MONDAY:	7 miles easy
TUESDAY:	2 mile warm-up; 10 × hill; 2 mile cooldown
WEDNESDAY:	4 miles easy or off
THURSDAY:	2 mile warm-up; 40-minute tempo run; 2 mile cooldown
FRIDAY:	4 miles easy or off
SATURDAY:	10 miles easy
SUNDAY:	off

Strength Work

	Week 11
MONDAY:	7 miles easy
TUESDAY:	2 mile warm-up; 12 × hill; 2 mile cooldown
WEDNESDAY:	4 miles easy or off
THURSDAY:	2 mile warm-up; 40-minute tempo run; 2 mile cooldown
FRIDAY:	4 miles easy or off
SATURDAY:	10 miles easy
SUNDAY:	off

The Half Marathon

THE 1:50 HALF MARATHON

To run a half marathon in 1 hour and 50 minutes you need to average 8 minutes and 23 seconds per mile.

Week 12

Track Work

MONDAY:	7 miles easy
TUESDAY:	1 mile warm-up, plus 4 striders; 4 × 1 mile in 8:13; 1 mile cooldown
WEDNESDAY:	4 miles easy or off
THURSDAY:	1 mile warm-up, plus 4 striders; 2 × 2 miles in 16:46; 1 mile cooldown
FRIDAY:	4 miles easy or off
SATURDAY:	12 miles easy
SUNDAY:	off

Week 13

Track Work

MONDAY:	7 miles easy
TUESDAY:	1 mile warm-up, plus 4 striders; 6 × 1 mile in 8:13; 1 mile cooldown
WEDNESDAY:	4 miles easy or off
THURSDAY:	1 mile warm-up, plus 4 striders; 3 × 2 miles in 16:46; 1 mile cooldown
FRIDAY:	4 miles easy or off
SATURDAY:	10 miles easy
SUNDAY:	off

Week 14

Track Work

MONDAY:	7 miles easy
TUESDAY:	1 mile warm-up, plus 4 striders; 6 × 1 mile in 8:13; 1 mile cooldown
WEDNESDAY:	4 miles easy or off
THURSDAY:	1 mile warm-up, plus 4 striders; 3 × 2 miles in 16:46; 1 mile cooldown
FRIDAY:	4 miles easy or off
SATURDAY:	12 miles easy
SUNDAY:	off

The Half Marathon

Track Work

Week 15		
	MONDAY:	7 miles easy
	TUESDAY:	1 mile warm-up, plus 4 striders; 6 × 1 mile in 8:13; 1 mile cooldown
	WEDNESDAY:	4 miles easy or off
	THURSDAY:	1 mile warm-up, plus 4 striders; 2 × 3 miles in 25:09; 1 mile cooldown
	FRIDAY:	4 miles easy or off
	SATURDAY:	12 miles easy
	SUNDAY:	off

Track Work

Week 16		
	MONDAY:	7 miles easy
	TUESDAY:	1 mile warm-up, plus 4 striders; 3 miles in 25:09, 2 miles in 16:26, 1 mile in 8:03; 1 mile cooldown
	WEDNESDAY:	4 miles easy or off
	THURSDAY:	1 mile warm-up, plus 4 striders; 4 miles in 33:32; 1 mile cooldown
	FRIDAY:	4 miles easy or off
	SATURDAY:	8 miles easy
	SUNDAY:	off

Track Work

Race Week		
	MONDAY:	6 miles easy
	TUESDAY:	1 mile warm-up, plus 4 striders; 3 × 800 in 4:12; 1 mile cooldown
	WEDNESDAY:	off
	THURSDAY:	off
	FRIDAY:	3 miles easy
	SATURDAY:	RACE
	SUNDAY:	Rest, recover, and celebrate

The Half Marathon

THE 2:00 HALF MARATHON

To run a half marathon in 2 hours you need to average 9 minutes and 9 seconds per mile.

Week 12

Track Work

MONDAY:	7 miles easy
TUESDAY:	1 mile warm-up, plus 4 striders; 4 × 1 mile in 8:59; 1 mile cooldown
WEDNESDAY:	4 miles easy or off
THURSDAY:	1 mile warm-up, plus 4 striders; 2 × 2 miles in 18:18; 1 mile cooldown
FRIDAY:	4 miles easy or off
SATURDAY:	10 miles easy
SUNDAY:	off

Week 13

Track Work

MONDAY:	7 miles easy
TUESDAY:	1 mile warm-up, plus 4 striders; 6 × 1 mile in 8:59; 1 mile cooldown
WEDNESDAY:	4 miles easy or off
THURSDAY:	1 mile warm-up, plus 4 striders; 3 × 2 miles in 18:18; 1 mile cooldown
FRIDAY:	4 miles easy or off
SATURDAY:	12 miles easy
SUNDAY:	off

Week 14

Track Work

MONDAY:	7 miles easy
TUESDAY:	1 mile warm-up, plus 4 striders; 6 × 1 mile in 8:59; 1 mile cooldown
WEDNESDAY:	4 miles easy or off
THURSDAY:	1 mile warm-up, plus 4 striders; 3 × 2 miles in 18:18; 1 mile cooldown
FRIDAY:	4 miles easy or off
SATURDAY:	10 miles easy
SUNDAY:	off

The Half Marathon

Week 15

Track Work

MONDAY:	7 miles easy
TUESDAY:	1 mile warm-up, plus 4 striders; 6 × 1 mile in 8:59; 1 mile cooldown
WEDNESDAY:	4 miles easy or off
THURSDAY:	1 mile warm-up, plus 4 striders; 2 × 3 miles in 27:27; 1 mile cooldown
FRIDAY:	4 miles easy or off
SATURDAY:	12 miles easy
SUNDAY:	off

Week 16

Track Work

MONDAY:	7 miles easy
TUESDAY:	1 mile warm-up, plus 4 striders; 3 miles in 27:27, 2 miles in 18:08, 1 mile in 8:59; 1 mile cooldown
WEDNESDAY:	4 miles easy or off
THURSDAY:	1 mile warm-up, plus 4 striders; 4 miles in 36:36; 1 mile cooldown
FRIDAY:	4 miles easy or off
SATURDAY:	8 miles easy
SUNDAY:	off

Race Week

Track Work

MONDAY:	6 miles easy
TUESDAY:	1 mile warm-up, plus 4 striders; 3 × 800 in 4:34; 1 mile cooldown
WEDNESDAY:	off
THURSDAY:	off
FRIDAY:	3 miles easy
SATURDAY:	RACE
SUNDAY:	Rest, recover, and celebrate

The Half Marathon

THE 2:10 HALF MARATHON

To run a half marathon in 2 hours and 10 minutes you need to average 9 minutes and 55 seconds per mile.

Track Work

Week 12		
	MONDAY:	7 miles easy
	TUESDAY:	1 mile warm-up, plus 4 striders; 4 × 1 mile in 9:45; 1 mile cooldown
	WEDNESDAY:	4 miles easy or off
	THURSDAY:	1 mile warm-up, plus 4 striders; 2 × 2 miles in 19:50; 1 mile cooldown
	FRIDAY:	4 miles easy or off
	SATURDAY:	10 miles easy
	SUNDAY:	off

Track Work

Week 13		
	MONDAY:	7 miles easy
	TUESDAY:	1 mile warm-up, plus 4 striders; 6 × 1 mile in 9:45; 1 mile cooldown
	WEDNESDAY:	4 miles easy or off
	THURSDAY:	1 mile warm-up, plus 4 striders; 3 × 2 miles in 19:50; 1 mile cooldown
	FRIDAY:	4 miles easy or off
	SATURDAY:	12 miles easy
	SUNDAY:	off

Track Work

Week 14		
	MONDAY:	7 miles easy
	TUESDAY:	1 mile warm-up, plus 4 striders; 6 × 1 mile in 9:45; 1 mile cooldown
	WEDNESDAY:	4 miles easy or off
	THURSDAY:	1 mile warm-up, plus 4 striders; 3 × 2 miles in 19:50; 1 mile cooldown
	FRIDAY:	4 miles easy or off
	SATURDAY:	10 miles easy
	SUNDAY:	off

The Half Marathon

Track Work

MONDAY:	7 miles easy
TUESDAY:	1 mile warm-up, plus 4 striders; 6 × 1 mile in 9:45; 1 mile cooldown
WEDNESDAY:	4 miles easy or off
THURSDAY:	1 mile warm-up, plus 4 striders; 2 × 3 miles in 29:45; 1 mile cooldown
FRIDAY:	4 miles easy or off
SATURDAY:	12 miles easy
SUNDAY:	off

Track Work

MONDAY:	7 miles easy
TUESDAY:	1 mile warm-up, plus 4 striders; 3 miles in 29:45, 2 miles in 19:30, 1 mile in 9:30; 1 mile cooldown
WEDNESDAY:	4 miles easy or off
THURSDAY:	1 mile warm-up, plus 4 striders; 4 miles in 39:35; 1 mile cooldown
FRIDAY:	4 miles easy or off
SATURDAY:	8 miles easy
SUNDAY:	off

Track Work

MONDAY:	6 miles easy
TUESDAY:	1 mile warm-up, plus 4 striders; 3 × 800 in 4:27; 1 mile cooldown
WEDNESDAY:	off
THURSDAY:	off
FRIDAY:	3 miles easy
SATURDAY:	RACE
SUNDAY:	Rest, recover, and celebrate

The Half Marathon

THE 2:20 HALF MARATHON

To run a half marathon in 2 hours and 20 minutes you must average 10 minutes and 41 seconds per mile.

Track Work

Week 12		
	MONDAY:	7 miles easy
	TUESDAY:	1 mile warm-up, plus 4 striders; 4 × 1 mile in 10:31; 1 mile cooldown
	WEDNESDAY:	4 miles easy or off
	THURSDAY:	1 mile warm-up, plus 4 striders; 2 × 2 miles in 21:22; 1 mile cooldown
	FRIDAY:	4 miles easy or off
	SATURDAY:	10 miles easy
	SUNDAY:	off

Track Work

Week 13		
	MONDAY:	7 miles easy
	TUESDAY:	1 mile warm-up, plus 4 striders; 6 × 1 mile in 10:31; 1 mile cooldown
	WEDNESDAY:	4 miles easy or off
	THURSDAY:	1 mile warm-up, plus 4 striders; 3 × 2 miles in 21:22; 1 mile cooldown
	FRIDAY:	4 miles easy or off
	SATURDAY:	12 miles easy
	SUNDAY:	off

Track Work

Week 14		
	MONDAY:	7 miles easy
	TUESDAY:	1 mile warm-up, plus 4 striders; 6 × 1 mile in 10:31; 1 mile cooldown
	WEDNESDAY:	4 miles easy or off
	THURSDAY:	1 mile warm-up, plus 4 striders; 3 × 2 miles in 21:22; 1 mile cooldown
	FRIDAY:	4 miles easy or off
	SATURDAY:	10 miles easy
	SUNDAY:	off

The Half Marathon

Week 15

Track Work

MONDAY:	7 miles easy
TUESDAY:	1 mile warm-up, plus 4 striders; 6 × 1 mile in 10:31; 1 mile cooldown
WEDNESDAY:	4 miles easy
THURSDAY:	1 mile warm-up, plus 4 striders; 2 × 3 miles in 32:03; 1 mile cooldown
FRIDAY:	4 miles easy or off
SATURDAY:	12 miles easy
SUNDAY:	off

Week 16

Track Work

MONDAY:	7 miles easy
TUESDAY:	1 mile warm-up, plus 4 striders; 3 miles in 32:03, 2 miles in 21:02, 1 mile in 10:11; 1 mile cooldown
WEDNESDAY:	4 miles easy or off
THURSDAY:	1 mile warm-up, plus 4 striders; 4 miles in 42:44; 1 mile cooldown
FRIDAY:	4 miles easy or off
SATURDAY:	8 miles easy
SUNDAY:	off

Race Week

Track Work

MONDAY:	6 miles easy
TUESDAY:	1 mile warm-up, plus 4 striders; 3 × 800 in 5:20; 1 mile cooldown
WEDNESDAY:	off
THURSDAY:	off
FRIDAY:	3 miles easy
SATURDAY:	RACE
SUNDAY:	Rest, recover, and celebrate

The Half Marathon

THE MARATHON
Road Work and Track Work for all marathon training schedules

Road Work

<table>
<tr><td rowspan="7">Week 1</td><td>MONDAY:</td><td>6 miles easy</td></tr>
<tr><td>TUESDAY:</td><td>5 miles easy</td></tr>
<tr><td>WEDNESDAY:</td><td>8 miles easy</td></tr>
<tr><td>THURSDAY:</td><td>4 miles easy or off</td></tr>
<tr><td>FRIDAY:</td><td>6 miles easy</td></tr>
<tr><td>SATURDAY:</td><td>10 miles easy</td></tr>
<tr><td>SUNDAY:</td><td>off</td></tr>
</table>

Road Work

<table>
<tr><td rowspan="7">Week 2</td><td>MONDAY:</td><td>6 miles easy</td></tr>
<tr><td>TUESDAY:</td><td>6 miles easy</td></tr>
<tr><td>WEDNESDAY:</td><td>8 miles easy</td></tr>
<tr><td>THURSDAY:</td><td>4 miles easy or off</td></tr>
<tr><td>FRIDAY:</td><td>6 miles easy</td></tr>
<tr><td>SATURDAY:</td><td>12 miles easy</td></tr>
<tr><td>SUNDAY:</td><td>off</td></tr>
</table>

Road Work

<table>
<tr><td rowspan="7">Week 3</td><td>MONDAY:</td><td>6 miles easy</td></tr>
<tr><td>TUESDAY:</td><td>6 miles easy</td></tr>
<tr><td>WEDNESDAY:</td><td>10 miles easy</td></tr>
<tr><td>THURSDAY:</td><td>4 miles easy or off</td></tr>
<tr><td>FRIDAY:</td><td>6 miles easy</td></tr>
<tr><td>SATURDAY:</td><td>10 miles easy</td></tr>
<tr><td>SUNDAY:</td><td>off</td></tr>
</table>

Road Work

<table>
<tr><td rowspan="7">Week 4</td><td>MONDAY:</td><td>6 miles easy</td></tr>
<tr><td>TUESDAY:</td><td>6 miles easy; 6 striders</td></tr>
<tr><td>WEDNESDAY:</td><td>10 miles easy</td></tr>
<tr><td>THURSDAY:</td><td>4 miles easy or off</td></tr>
<tr><td>FRIDAY:</td><td>6 miles easy; 6 striders</td></tr>
<tr><td>SATURDAY:</td><td>14 miles easy</td></tr>
<tr><td>SUNDAY:</td><td>off</td></tr>
</table>

The Marathon

Week 5

Road Work

MONDAY:	6 miles easy
TUESDAY:	6 miles easy; 6 striders
WEDNESDAY:	10 miles easy
THURSDAY:	4 miles easy or off
FRIDAY:	5 miles easy; 6 striders
SATURDAY:	16 miles easy
SUNDAY:	off

Week 6

Road Work

MONDAY:	6 miles easy
TUESDAY:	6 miles easy; 8 striders
WEDNESDAY:	10 miles easy
THURSDAY:	4 miles easy or off
FRIDAY:	5 miles easy; 8 striders
SATURDAY:	12 miles easy
SUNDAY:	off

Week 7

Road Work

MONDAY:	6 miles easy
TUESDAY:	6 miles easy; 8 striders
WEDNESDAY:	10 miles easy
THURSDAY:	4 miles easy or off
FRIDAY:	5 miles easy; 8 striders
SATURDAY:	18 miles easy
SUNDAY:	off

Week 8

Road Work

MONDAY:	6 miles easy
TUESDAY:	6 miles easy; 8 striders
WEDNESDAY:	10 miles easy
THURSDAY:	4 miles easy or off
FRIDAY:	5 miles easy; 8 striders
SATURDAY:	20 miles easy
SUNDAY:	off

The Marathon

Strength Work

<table>
<tbody>
<tr><td rowspan="7">Week 9</td><td>MONDAY:</td><td>6 miles easy</td></tr>
<tr><td>TUESDAY:</td><td>6 miles easy</td></tr>
<tr><td>WEDNESDAY:</td><td>2 mile warm-up; 40-minute tempo run; 2 mile cooldown</td></tr>
<tr><td>THURSDAY:</td><td>4 miles easy or off</td></tr>
<tr><td>FRIDAY:</td><td>5 miles easy</td></tr>
<tr><td>SATURDAY:</td><td>16 miles easy</td></tr>
<tr><td>SUNDAY:</td><td>off</td></tr>
</tbody>
</table>

Strength Work

<table>
<tbody>
<tr><td rowspan="7">Week 10</td><td>MONDAY:</td><td>6 miles easy</td></tr>
<tr><td>TUESDAY:</td><td>6 miles easy</td></tr>
<tr><td>WEDNESDAY:</td><td>2 mile warm-up; 40-minute tempo run; 2 mile cooldown</td></tr>
<tr><td>THURSDAY:</td><td>4 miles easy or off</td></tr>
<tr><td>FRIDAY:</td><td>5 miles easy</td></tr>
<tr><td>SATURDAY:</td><td>20 miles easy</td></tr>
<tr><td>SUNDAY:</td><td>off</td></tr>
</tbody>
</table>

Strength Work

<table>
<tbody>
<tr><td rowspan="7">Week 11</td><td>MONDAY:</td><td>6 miles easy</td></tr>
<tr><td>TUESDAY:</td><td>6 miles easy</td></tr>
<tr><td>WEDNESDAY:</td><td>2 mile warm-up; 40-minute tempo run; 2 mile cooldown</td></tr>
<tr><td>THURSDAY:</td><td>4 miles easy or off</td></tr>
<tr><td>FRIDAY:</td><td>5 miles easy</td></tr>
<tr><td>SATURDAY:</td><td>12 miles easy</td></tr>
<tr><td>SUNDAY:</td><td>off</td></tr>
</tbody>
</table>

The Marathon

THE 4:00 MARATHON

To run a marathon in 4 hours you need to average 9 minutes and 9 seconds per mile. But you will target 8:59 pace for your race. (This is because you can't hold race pace for 26.2 miles.)

Track Work

Week 12		
	MONDAY:	6 miles easy
	TUESDAY:	6 miles easy
	WEDNESDAY:	1 mile warm-up, plus 4 striders; 6 × 1 mile in 8:59; 1 mile cooldown
	THURSDAY:	4 miles easy or off
	FRIDAY:	5 miles easy
	SATURDAY:	20 miles easy
	SUNDAY:	off

Track Work

Week 13		
	MONDAY:	6 miles easy
	TUESDAY:	6 miles easy
	WEDNESDAY:	1 mile warm-up, plus 4 striders; 8 × 1 mile in 8:59; 1 mile cooldown
	THURSDAY:	4 miles easy or off
	FRIDAY:	5 miles easy
	SATURDAY:	12 miles easy
	SUNDAY:	off

Track Work

Week 14		
	MONDAY:	6 miles easy
	TUESDAY:	6 miles easy
	WEDNESDAY:	1 mile warm-up, plus 4 striders; 4 × 2 miles in 17:58; 1 mile cooldown
	THURSDAY:	4 miles easy or off
	FRIDAY:	5 miles easy
	SATURDAY:	22 miles easy
	SUNDAY:	off

The Marathon

Track Work

Week 15		
MONDAY:	6 miles easy
TUESDAY:	off
WEDNESDAY:	6 miles easy
THURSDAY:	4 miles easy or off
FRIDAY:	5 miles easy
SATURDAY:	1 mile warm-up; 4 miles at marathon pace; 4 miles on the track at 8:49 per mile; 4 miles at marathon pace; 1 mile cooldown
SUNDAY:	off

Track Work

Week 16		
MONDAY:	6 miles easy
TUESDAY:	off
WEDNESDAY:	6 miles easy
THURSDAY:	off
FRIDAY:	5 miles easy
SATURDAY:	1 mile warm-up; 8 miles at marathon pace; 1 mile cooldown
SUNDAY:	off

Track Work

Race Week		
MONDAY:	5 miles easy
TUESDAY:	3 miles at marathon pace
WEDNESDAY:	off
THURSDAY:	off
FRIDAY:	3 miles easy
SATURDAY:	RACE
SUNDAY:	Rest, recover, and celebrate

The Marathon

THE 4:15 MARATHON

To run a marathon in 4 hours and 15 minutes you need to average 9 minutes and 43 seconds per mile. But you will target 9:33 for your race. (This is because you can't hold race pace for 26.2 miles.)

Track Work

Week 12		
MONDAY:	6 miles easy
TUESDAY:	6 miles easy
WEDNESDAY:	1 mile warm-up, plus 4 striders; 6 × 1 mile in 9:33; 1 mile cooldown
THURSDAY:	4 miles easy or off
FRIDAY:	5 miles easy
SATURDAY:	20 miles easy
SUNDAY:	off

Track Work

Week 13		
MONDAY:	6 miles easy
TUESDAY:	6 miles easy
WEDNESDAY:	1 mile warm-up, plus 4 striders; 8 × 1 mile in 9:33; 1 mile cooldown
THURSDAY:	4 miles easy or off
FRIDAY:	5 miles easy
SATURDAY:	12 miles easy
SUNDAY:	off

Track Work

Week 14		
MONDAY:	6 miles easy
TUESDAY:	6 miles easy
WEDNESDAY:	1 mile warm-up, plus 4 striders; 4 × 2 miles in 19:06; 1 mile cooldown
THURSDAY:	4 miles easy or off
FRIDAY:	5 miles easy
SATURDAY:	22 miles easy
SUNDAY:	off

Track Work

Week 15

MONDAY:	6 miles easy
TUESDAY:	off
WEDNESDAY:	6 miles easy
THURSDAY:	4 miles easy or off
FRIDAY:	5 miles easy
SATURDAY:	1 mile warm-up; 4 miles at marathon pace; 4 miles on the track at 9:23 per mile; 4 miles at marathon pace; 1 mile cooldown
SUNDAY:	off

Track Work

Week 16

MONDAY:	6 miles easy
TUESDAY:	off
WEDNESDAY:	6 miles easy
THURSDAY:	off
FRIDAY:	5 miles easy
SATURDAY:	1 mile warm-up; 8 miles at marathon pace; 1 mile cooldown
SUNDAY:	off

Track Work

Race Week

MONDAY:	5 miles easy
TUESDAY:	3 miles at marathon pace
WEDNESDAY:	off
THURSDAY:	off
FRIDAY:	3 miles easy
SATURDAY:	RACE
SUNDAY:	Rest, recover, and celebrate

The Marathon

THE 4:30 MARATHON

To run a marathon in 4 hours and 30 minutes you need to average 10 minutes and 17 seconds per mile. But you will target 10:07 for your race. (This is because you can't hold race pace for 26.2 miles.)

Track Work

Week 12		
	MONDAY:	6 miles easy
	TUESDAY:	6 miles easy
	WEDNESDAY:	1 mile warm-up, plus 4 striders; 6 × 1 mile in 10:07; 1 mile cooldown
	THURSDAY:	4 miles easy or off
	FRIDAY:	5 miles easy
	SATURDAY:	20 miles easy
	SUNDAY:	off

Track Work

Week 13		
	MONDAY:	6 miles easy
	TUESDAY:	6 miles easy
	WEDNESDAY:	1 mile warm-up, plus 4 striders; 8 × 1 mile in 10:07; 1 mile cooldown
	THURSDAY:	4 miles easy or off
	FRIDAY:	5 miles easy
	SATURDAY:	12 miles easy
	SUNDAY:	off

Track Work

Week 14		
	MONDAY:	6 miles easy
	TUESDAY:	6 miles easy
	WEDNESDAY:	1 mile warm-up, plus 4 striders; 4 × 2 miles in 20:14; 1 mile cooldown
	THURSDAY:	4 miles easy or off
	FRIDAY:	5 miles easy
	SATURDAY:	22 miles
	SUNDAY:	off

The Marathon

Track Work

Week 15	**MONDAY:**	6 miles easy
	TUESDAY:	off
	WEDNESDAY:	6 miles easy
	THURSDAY:	off
	FRIDAY:	5 miles easy
	SATURDAY:	1 mile warm-up, 4 miles at marathon pace; 4 miles on the track in 9:57 per mile; 4 miles at marathon pace; 1 mile cooldown
	SUNDAY:	off

Track Work

Week 16	**MONDAY:**	6 miles easy
	TUESDAY:	off
	WEDNESDAY:	6 miles easy
	THURSDAY:	off
	FRIDAY:	5 miles easy
	SATURDAY:	1 mile warm-up; 8 miles at marathon pace; 1 mile cooldown
	SUNDAY:	off

Track Work

Race Week	**MONDAY:**	5 miles easy
	TUESDAY:	3 miles at marathon pace
	WEDNESDAY:	off
	THURSDAY:	off
	FRIDAY:	3 miles easy
	SATURDAY:	RACE
	SUNDAY:	Rest, recover, and celebrate

The Marathon

THE 4:45 MARATHON

To run a marathon in 4 hours and 45 minutes you need to average 10 minutes and 52 seconds per mile. But you will target 10:42 per mile for your race. (This is because you can't hold race pace for 26.2 miles.)

Track Work

Week 12		
MONDAY:	6 miles easy
TUESDAY:	6 miles easy
WEDNESDAY:	1 mile warm-up, plus 4 striders; 6 × 1 mile in 10:42; 1 mile cooldown
THURSDAY:	4 miles easy or off
FRIDAY:	5 miles easy
SATURDAY:	20 miles easy
SUNDAY:	off

Track Work

Week 13		
MONDAY:	6 miles easy
TUESDAY:	6 miles easy
WEDNESDAY:	1 mile warm-up, plus 4 striders; 8 × 1 mile in 10:42; 1 mile cooldown
THURSDAY:	4 miles easy or off
FRIDAY:	5 miles easy
SATURDAY:	12 miles easy
SUNDAY:	off

Track Work

Week 14		
MONDAY:	6 miles easy
TUESDAY:	6 miles easy
WEDNESDAY:	1 mile warm-up, plus 4 striders; 4 × 2 miles in 21:24; 1 mile cooldown
THURSDAY:	4 miles easy or off
FRIDAY:	5 miles easy
SATURDAY:	22 miles easy
SUNDAY:	off

The Marathon

Track Work

Week 15		
MONDAY:	6 miles easy	
TUESDAY:	off	
WEDNESDAY:	6 miles easy	
THURSDAY:	off	
FRIDAY:	5 miles easy	
SATURDAY:	1 mile warm-up; 4 miles at marathon pace; 4 miles on the track in 10:32 per mile; 4 miles at marathon pace; 1 mile cooldown	
SUNDAY:	off	

Track Work

Week 16		
MONDAY:	6 miles easy	
TUESDAY:	off	
WEDNESDAY:	6 miles easy	
THURSDAY:	off	
FRIDAY:	5 miles easy	
SATURDAY:	1 mile warm-up; 8 miles at marathon pace; 1 mile cooldown	
SUNDAY:	off	

Track Work

Race Week		
MONDAY:	5 miles easy	
TUESDAY:	3 miles at marathon pace	
WEDNESDAY:	off	
THURSDAY:	off	
FRIDAY:	3 miles easy	
SATURDAY:	RACE	
SUNDAY:	Rest, recover, and celebrate	

The Marathon

CHAPTER 7

The Training Log

WEEK 1: ROAD WORK

All journeys begin with first steps. Make your first steps strong and confident.

Monday

Workout:

Weather:

How did it go: _____
_____
_____

Tuesday

Workout:

Weather:

How did it go: _____
_____
_____

Wednesday

Workout:

Weather:

How did it go: _____
_____
_____

Thursday

Workout:

Weather:

How did it go: _____
_____
_____

Road Work

Friday

Workout:

Weather:

How did it go: _____
_____
_____

Saturday

Workout:

Weather:

How did it go: _____
_____
_____

Week in Review

Workout:

Weather:

How did it go: _____
_____
_____
_____
_____
_____
_____

Road Work

"The will to win means nothing without the will to prepare."
—JUMA IKANGAA, ELITE MARATHONER

WEEK 2: ROAD WORK

Believe it or not, week two is a make-or-break moment for many people starting a running program. So make it through week two and you are on your way.

Monday

Workout:

Weather:

How did it go: _____
_____
_____

Tuesday

Workout:

Weather:

How did it go: _____
_____
_____

Wednesday

Workout:

Weather:

How did it go: _____
_____
_____

Thursday

Workout:

Weather:

How did it go: _____
_____
_____

Road Work

Friday

Workout:

Weather:

How did it go: _____
_____
_____

Saturday

Workout:

Weather:

How did it go: _____
_____
_____

Week in Review

Workout:

Weather:

How did it go: _____
_____
_____
_____
_____
_____
_____

Road Work

"If one can stick to the training throughout the many long years, then willpower is no longer a problem."
—EMIL ZATOPEK, OLYMPIC CHAMPION

WEEK 3: ROAD WORK

Remember to take the "talk test" when you are running easy. If you can't carry on a conversation while running, you are running too fast.

Monday

Workout:

Weather:

How did it go: _____
_____
_____

Tuesday

Workout:

Weather:

How did it go: _____
_____
_____

Wednesday

Workout:

Weather:

How did it go: _____
_____
_____

Thursday

Workout:

Weather:

How did it go: _____
_____
_____

Road Work

Friday

Workout:

Weather:

How did it go: _____

_____

_____

Saturday

Workout:

Weather:

How did it go: _____

_____

_____

Week in Review

Workout:

Weather:

How did it go: _____

_____

_____

_____

_____

_____

_____

Road Work

"Good things come slow—especially in distance running."
—BILL DELLINGER, OLYMPIC MEDALIST AND COACH

WEEK 4: ROAD WORK

The key to any training program is consistency. Make it your goal to stay consistent—nail each training day as planned—as you round out your first month of training.

Monday

Workout:

Weather:

How did it go: _____
_____
_____

Tuesday

Workout:

Weather:

How did it go: _____
_____
_____

Wednesday

Workout:

Weather:

How did it go: _____
_____
_____

Thursday

Workout:

Weather:

How did it go: _____
_____
_____

Road Work

Friday

Workout:

Weather:

How did it go: _____
_____
_____

Saturday

Workout:

Weather:

How did it go: _____
_____
_____

Week in Review

Workout:

Weather:

How did it go: _____
_____
_____
_____
_____
_____
_____

Road Work

"Long-distance running is particularly good training in perseverance."
—MAO TSE-TUNG

WEEK 5: ROAD WORK

Endurance is earned through miles of sweat.

<table>
<tr><td>Monday</td><td>Workout:

Weather:

How did it go: _____
_____
_____</td></tr>
</table>

Monday

Workout:

Weather:

How did it go: _____
_____
_____

Tuesday

Workout:

Weather:

How did it go: _____
_____
_____

Wednesday

Workout:

Weather:

How did it go: _____
_____
_____

Thursday

Workout:

Weather:

How did it go: _____
_____
_____

Road Work

Friday

Workout:

Weather:

How did it go: _____
_____
_____

Saturday

Workout:

Weather:

How did it go: _____
_____
_____

Week in Review

Workout:

Weather:

How did it go: _____
_____
_____
_____
_____
_____
_____

Road Work

"The long run is what puts the tiger in the cat."
—BILL SQUIRES, COACH

WEEK 6: ROAD WORK

Be fresh—mentally and physically—for your Saturday long run by making Friday a total recovery run.

Monday

Workout:

Weather:

How did it go: _____
_____
_____

Tuesday

Workout:

Weather:

How did it go: _____
_____
_____

Wednesday

Workout:

Weather:

How did it go: _____
_____
_____

Thursday

Workout:

Weather:

How did it go: _____
_____
_____

Road Work

Friday

Workout:

Weather:

How did it go: _____
_____
_____

Saturday

Workout:

Weather:

How did it go: _____
_____
_____

Week in Review

Workout:

Weather:

How did it go: _____
_____
_____
_____
_____
_____
_____

Road Work

"Training is principally an act of faith."
—FRANZ STAMPFL, COACH

WEEK 7: ROAD WORK

Shaking out your arms midway through a run is a great way to stay loose.

Monday

Workout:

Weather:

How did it go: _____
_____
_____

Tuesday

Workout:

Weather:

How did it go: _____
_____
_____

Wednesday

Workout:

Weather:

How did it go: _____
_____
_____

Thursday

Workout:

Weather:

How did it go: _____
_____
_____

Road Work

Friday

Workout:

Weather:

How did it go: _____
_____
_____

Saturday

Workout:

Weather:

How did it go: _____
_____
_____

Week in Review

Workout:

Weather:

How did it go: _____
_____
_____
_____
_____
_____
_____
_____

"Workouts are like brushing my teeth: I don't think about them,
I just do them."
—PATTI SUE PLUMER, U.S. OLYMPIAN

Road Work

WEEK 8: ROAD WORK

Cap off two months of Road Work with your favorite meal on Sunday.

Monday

Workout:

Weather:

How did it go: _____
_____
_____

Tuesday

Workout:

Weather:

How did it go: _____
_____
_____

Wednesday

Workout:

Weather:

How did it go: _____
_____
_____

Thursday

Workout:

Weather:

How did it go: _____
_____
_____

Road Work

Friday

Workout:

Weather:

How did it go: _____
_____
_____

Saturday

Workout:

Weather:

How did it go: _____
_____
_____

Week in Review

Workout:

Weather:

How did it go: _____
_____
_____
_____
_____
_____
_____
_____

"If you put down a good, solid foundation and build one room after another,
pretty soon you have a house."
—ROD DIXON, NEW YORK CITY MARATHON WINNER

Road Work

WEEK 9: STRENGTH WORK

Start any hill workout or any tempo run gradually. Then work up to pace.

Monday

Workout:

Weather:

How did it go: _____
_____
_____

Tuesday

Workout:

Weather:

How did it go: _____
_____
_____

Wednesday

Workout:

Weather:

How did it go: _____
_____
_____

Thursday

Workout:

Weather:

How did it go: _____
_____
_____

Strength Work

Friday

Workout:

Weather:

How did it go: _____
_____
_____

Saturday

Workout:

Weather:

How did it go: _____
_____
_____

Week in Review

Workout:

Weather:

How did it go: _____
_____
_____
_____
_____
_____
_____

Strength Work

"Everyone is an athlete. The only difference is that some of us are in training, and some are not."
—DR. GEORGE SHEEHAN, AUTHOR AND RUNNING PHILOSOPHER

WEEK 10: STRENGTH WORK

There is "strength" in numbers. The most important hill is the last one. The most important minute of your tempo run is the last one.

Monday

Workout:

Weather:

How did it go: _____
_____
_____

Tuesday

Workout:

Weather:

How did it go: _____
_____
_____

Wednesday

Workout:

Weather:

How did it go: _____
_____
_____

Thursday

Workout:

Weather:

How did it go: _____
_____
_____

Strength Work

Friday

Workout:

Weather:

How did it go: _____
_____
_____

Saturday

Workout:

Weather:

How did it go: _____
_____
_____

Week in Review

Workout:

Weather:

How did it go: _____
_____
_____
_____
_____
_____
_____

Strength Work

"Overtraining is the biggest problem incurred by runners who lack the experience or discipline to cope with their own enthusiasm."
—MARTY LIQUORI, U.S. OLYMPIAN

WEEK 11: STRENGTH WORK

Make sleep a priority this week; when you wake up you will be stronger.

Monday

Workout:

Weather:

How did it go: _____
_____
_____

Tuesday

Workout:

Weather:

How did it go: _____
_____
_____

Wednesday

Workout:

Weather:

How did it go: _____
_____
_____

Thursday

Workout:

Weather:

How did it go: _____
_____
_____

Strength Work

Friday

Workout:

Weather:

How did it go: _____
_____
_____

Saturday

Workout:

Weather:

How did it go: _____
_____
_____

Week in Review

Workout:

Weather:

How did it go: _____
_____
_____
_____
_____
_____
_____

Strength Work

"Train, don't strain."
—RUNNING PROVERB

WEEK 12: TRACK WORK

Meet your training partner at the track this week for some mutual support.

Monday

Workout:

Weather:

How did it go: _____
_____
_____

Tuesday

Workout:

Weather:

How did it go: _____
_____
_____

Wednesday

Workout:

Weather:

How did it go: _____
_____
_____

Thursday

Workout:

Weather:

How did it go: _____
_____
_____

Track Work

Friday

Workout:

Weather:

How did it go: _____
_____
_____

Saturday

Workout:

Weather:

How did it go: _____
_____
_____

Week in Review

Workout:

Weather:

How did it go: _____
_____
_____
_____
_____
_____
_____

Track Work

*"You find out by trial and error what the optimal level of training is.
If I found I was training too hard, I would drop it back for a day or two."*
—SIR ROGER BANNISTER, THE FIRST MAN TO BREAK THE FOUR-MINUTE MILE

WEEK 13: TRACK WORK

Don't neglect your warm-up or cooldown. They help you prepare and recover.

Monday

Workout:

Weather:

How did it go: _____
_____
_____

Tuesday

Workout:

Weather:

How did it go: _____
_____
_____

Wednesday

Workout:

Weather:

How did it go: _____
_____
_____

Thursday

Workout:

Weather:

How did it go: _____
_____
_____

Track Work

Friday

Workout:

Weather:

How did it go: _____
_____
_____
_____

Saturday

Workout:

Weather:

How did it go: _____
_____
_____
_____

Week in Review

Workout:

Weather:

How did it go: _____
_____
_____
_____
_____
_____
_____
_____

Track Work

"The difference between a jogger and a runner is an entry blank."
—DR. GEORGE SHEEHAN

WEEK 14: TRACK WORK

Pace is crucial to any track workout. It makes sure you are not going too slow—or too fast.

Monday

Workout:

Weather:

How did it go: _____
_____
_____

Tuesday

Workout:

Weather:

How did it go: _____
_____
_____

Wednesday

Workout:

Weather:

How did it go: _____
_____
_____

Thursday

Workout:

Weather:

How did it go: _____
_____
_____

Track Work

Friday

Workout:

Weather:

How did it go: _____
_____
_____

Saturday

Workout:

Weather:

How did it go: _____
_____
_____

Week in Review

Workout:

Weather:

How did it go: _____
_____
_____
_____
_____
_____
_____

"Running is the greatest metaphor for life, because you get out of it
what you put into it."
—OPRAH WINFREY

Track Work

WEEK 15: TRACK WORK

Two weeks to go. Make each run count.

Monday

Workout:

Weather:

How did it go: _____
_____
_____

Tuesday

Workout:

Weather:

How did it go: _____
_____
_____

Wednesday

Workout:

Weather:

How did it go: _____
_____
_____

Thursday

Workout:

Weather:

How did it go: _____
_____
_____

Track Work

Friday

Workout:

Weather:

How did it go: _____
_____
_____

Saturday

Workout:

Weather:

How did it go: _____
_____
_____

Week in Review

Workout:

Weather:

How did it go: _____
_____
_____
_____
_____
_____
_____

"My feeling is that any day I am too busy to run is a day that I am too busy."
—JOHN BRYANT, FORMER DEPUTY EDITOR OF THE *LONDON TIMES*

Track Work

WEEK 16: TRACK WORK

Resist the urge to run hard this week. Your work is done. "The hay," as famous running coach Bill Bowerman says in the movie *Without Limits*, "is in the barn."

Monday

Workout:

Weather:

How did it go: _____
_____
_____

Tuesday

Workout:

Weather:

How did it go: _____
_____
_____

Wednesday

Workout:

Weather:

How did it go: _____
_____
_____

Thursday

Workout:

Weather:

How did it go: _____
_____
_____

Track Work

Friday

Workout:

Weather:

How did it go: _____
_____
_____

Saturday

Workout:

Weather:

How did it go: _____
_____
_____

Week in Review

Workout:

Weather:

How did it go: _____
_____
_____
_____
_____
_____
_____

Track Work

"Racing teaches us to challenge ourselves. It teaches us to push beyond where we thought we could go. It helps us to find out what we are made of."
—PATTI SUE PLUMER, U.S. OLYMPIAN

RACE WEEK: TRACK WORK

Make every day a recovery day in your mind. Concentrate and prepare mentally for Saturday's race.

Monday

Workout:

Weather:

How did it go: _____
_____
_____

Tuesday

Workout:

Weather:

How did it go: _____
_____
_____

Wednesday

Workout:

Weather:

How did it go: _____
_____
_____

Thursday

Workout:

Weather:

How did it go: _____
_____
_____

Track Work

Friday

Workout:

Weather:

How did it go: _____
_____
_____

Saturday

Workout:

Weather:

How did it go: _____
_____
_____

Week in Review

Workout:

Weather:

How did it go: _____
_____
_____
_____
_____
_____
_____

"The race is not always to the swift, but to those who keep on running."
—NIKE RUNNING POSTER

Track Work

CHAPTER 8

Race Week and Beyond

R ace week is when you make your final physical and mental preparations for the race. It is also, of course, when your race occurs. And it is the beginning of your recovery from that race.

That's a lot to pack into a fragile seven days. I say fragile because at the end of sixteen weeks of smart and intense training, your race is like a piece of finished sculpture. (Now, all you have to do is transport it from one building to another, without breaking it, so it can go on display.)

To better get a handle on all the challenges associated with Race Week, I have broken it down into four segments: Monday through Thursday; the 24-hour period directly preceding the starting gun; the race itself; and the postrace period.

Let's take them one at a time.

Monday to Thursday: Caution

These are the days when you can take all the gains you have earned during those sixteen weeks of training, crumple them up into a ball, and throw them out the window.

I have seen runners who didn't know any better (and runners who should have known better) completely ruin their chances at PRs just a couple of days before the race.

And how did they do it? They went out for runs on Tuesday or Wednesday of that week—and those runs turned into races. The runs were invigorating, exciting, and they ran well (they were in great shape). But, then, when they showed up for their race Saturday morning, they found that their midweek "races" had taken more out of them than they realized. And soon after the gun this fact dawned on them with cold certainty. They had blown it.

To make sure you don't blow it, here is a cautionary discussion of some misconceptions that tend to creep up during Race Week:

I STILL NEED MORE SPEED (OR MILEAGE)

During Race Week, all runs should be easy except where noted in the training schedules. A Tuesday light track workout at race pace, for instance, is a good way to get the legs moving during Race Week. (But it is a light workout and over with soon.) The danger here is to doubt your training, think you are not fit, and try to squeeze one or more hard workouts into the limited time remaining. This could be a heavy track workout or, if you are training for a half marathon or marathon, one more long run six or seven days out.

This is foolish for two reasons: The first reason is that you will not have time to recover and so the workout will leave you fatigued on race day. The second is that any hard training takes a while to take effect—you need to recover and grow stronger to see the benefits—and a hard workout during Race Week will not even have enough time to "sink in."

Therefore, any hard running you do during Race Week should be thought of in this manner: You are tiring yourself out for nothing.

I NEED TO FAST TO BE FAST

You need to fuel yourself for your race, but as the race draws near the exact opposite impulse often strikes runners. They see a drop in mileage during the last week (or, for marathoners, during the last two weeks) as a reason to cut calories. They skimp on breakfast, nibble on lunch, and then skip dinner altogether. Because they are not running as much, they feel fat, and the only way to combat this feeling is to put less food in their mouths—which, of course, leads directly to a race where running PRs is simply out of the question, because they have not properly fueled themselves for their races.

During Race Week the lesson is simple: You need to eat. For starters, food keeps energy levels high (this, in turn, combats prerace anxiety). It also stores fuel (needed to get you to the finish line). And it aids in recovery (your body is repairing damaged muscle tissue from sixteen weeks of training). All three are critical for PR race success.

The easiest way, then, to ensure that you are getting enough food during Race Week is to continue to eat three meals each day. Your body should be conditioned to eat (and be hungry) at these times, so keep up the daily routine. Pay special attention to eating dinner, especially if you run during the late afternoon as cutting back (or cutting out) on a run at that time will lessen the usual predinnertime hunger and the motivation to eat.

If any food can be cut during Race Week, it should be the "reward snack," the large cookie that comes on the afternoon of your long run or the bowl of ice cream on the night of a hard track workout. Save that eating for after the race.

I DON'T NEED REST

Resting is vital because the only way you can be completely ready to run a PR is to be so rested you are bursting at the seams to race but at the same time also at your highest level of fitness. This is your final "peak" for the race, and it is a tricky thing. Your training program—Road Work, Strength Work, Track Work—has also been designed, over the course of months, to peak you for your race. So is the fact that in the weeks leading up to your race, you have been cutting back on mileage and the intensity of your workouts. But all that stuff has been the easy part. All you had to do was read a training program and then go out and do the prescribed workout.

How to Rest

Resting effectively close to race time is easier said than done. Here are some ways to help you rest wisely:

- Book It: Save that must-read novel for the last week of your training program.

- DVD Time: Catch up on the Oscar winners you failed to see. But go easy on the salty popcorn.

- Cup of Joe with Joe: Meet your training partner for a cup of coffee during the time you would regularly be running. Talk about your upcoming race.

- Nap Time for Yours Truly: Take some real downtime on the couch. Napping frequently as the race approaches is a great secret among elite runners.

- Study Up: Spend your normal running hour going over the race brochure and website. Just make sure not to wear your running shoes while doing this or you may be tempted to get up and run.

The real challenge comes when "rest" starts to appear more frequently in the training program (for instance, most programs have two days of rest in a row during the final week). By the time you get to that point in your training—with the race just around the corner—many runners are either too antsy ("I can't take a day off now, I'll lose fitness") or too excited ("I'm ready to go!") to refrain from running.

Yet rest is what you must do at this time if you want to PR. To do so, you need to remember that you won't "lose fitness" by taking days off close to your race. If you have followed the training program, the exact opposite will happen—you will gain fitness as the body takes its final rest before race time to repair itself and grow stronger. (This is the internal magic of peaking.) Second, all that energy and enthusiasm is certainly a good thing, but it needs to be harnessed. Think of yourself as a racehorse in a paddock. You need to wait for the race to officially begin before you use that energy for its intended purpose.

Finally, there *is* a danger even if you do refrain from running during your rest day. That danger is you take that day to do a bunch of things that keep you on your feet, like running errands or mowing the lawn. "Rest day" means no running. But it also means taking it easy, keeping your feet up, and relaxing. So watch this tendency to burn that running energy through a series of nonrunning activities on your rest day.

Friday to Saturday Morning:
The 24-Hour Countdown

Just like the week before your race is a crucial time to make or break your PR, so is the final 24 hours before the gun—but even more so. During this time any mistake (the wrong food, a brisk run) will be magnified because you have only a few hours to recover from those mistakes.

Therefore, here's a 24-hour countdown to race time that you can follow to keep on the straight and narrow:

24 HOURS OUT: Jog easy for a few miles during the time you will be racing tomorrow.

23 HOURS OUT: Eat a healthy and light breakfast.

22 HOURS OUT: Spend a good chunk of the morning reading the newspaper or a novel.

19 HOURS OUT: Have a carbohydrate-rich lunch. For many, it is better to get your carbs at lunch than during the evening. This lessens the chance of waking up bloated on race morning.

18 HOURS OUT: Nap time.

16 HOURS OUT: Arrange your race gear for tomorrow. Lay out your shorts, shirt, socks, shoes, race number, pins, chip, hat, and anything else you might be wearing for your race.

14 HOURS OUT: Have a healthy and light dinner.

12 HOURS OUT: Watch TV or a DVD. Caution: An action movie or thriller might not be a good bet at this time, since it can hype you up and keep you from getting to sleep.

10 HOURS OUT: Sleep. It might be fitful, since you have so much on the line in the morning, but stay in bed and relax. (Also, the previous night's sleep is often designated as your real sleep night before your race. But why focus on just one night? Aim to get a good night's sleep each night during Race Week.)

3 HOURS OUT: Wake. Shower. Breakfast, if needed. (See Race-Day Breakfast? on page 147.)

1 HOUR OUT: Arrive at the race. Warm up with light jogging, some stretching, and a few striders.

15 MINUTES OUT: Find a spot behind the starting line. Put your watch in the stopwatch mode.

10 MINUTES OUT: Go over race strategy.

1 MINUTE OUT: Take deep breaths and shake out your arms.

GO!

> ## New Is Not Necessarily Better
>
> The one general rule that applies to everything done during Race Week is to not try anything new. No new foods, no new workouts, no new shoes (that goes for everyday shoes, too), no new routines (except the ones involving rest). Really. The whole idea is to feel as comfortable as possible as you continue to rest up and prepare for your race. And you can't do this if you are bombarding yourself with new stimuli.

The Race

When the gun goes off, it is all about you. Fortunately, by this time, you will have two things going for you that race novices do not: a familiarity with the race distance and with the race pace.

These two things should give you a good shot at your PR. But if you want to increase the odds substantially, you need to keep a few general racing rules in mind, and also come up with a workable race strategy—one you have thought out in the weeks leading up to the race—that you can employ during the race. Here's what you need to know:

START CONTROLLED, FINISH STRONG

When the gun goes off, everyone's first impulse is to take off much faster than race pace. Call it nerves. Call it excitement. It is probably a little of both. Yet you must tame this impulse or risk losing precious energy at a point in the race that is essentially meaningless (who cares how fast you run the first 800 meters of your 5K or 2 miles of your half marathon?).

A good way to help stay controlled at the start is to line up back in the pack a bit (but not too far back) rather than on the front lines. The congestion in front of you will force you to go out under control so you will have to work up to race pace (which will empower you), rather than bolt out and then have to slow down to find race pace (which leaves you feeling tentative and out of sorts).

In the same vein, you want to finish the race strongly, but with a controlled strength. Finishing strong does not mean sprinting wildly for the last 100 meters, as so many runners do at races. This is a simple waste of energy, since a sprint over that distance can only earn you a few seconds off your finishing time (and besides, a sprint like that is usually guilt driven, following a huge drop-off in pace). Instead, take that same energy—you know it's there—and use it to fuel race pace over the final 800 meters of a 5K or the final 2 miles of a half marathon, and you have a much more efficient use of that energy. And a finishing time that's more likely to be a PR.

THINK OF YOUR RACE IN SEGMENTS

Try thinking of a marathon, or even a 5K, in its entirety, and the task gets a little overwhelming. ("I have to run 26.2 miles! Do you know how far that is from my house?" "I have to run 3 consecutive miles in 9 minutes per mile! Just one of those miles puts me in pain!") If you think of your race as a whole, you will lose sleep, have a hard time training, and fail utterly in your quest for a PR.

Instead, what you need to do is what you did with the training process—divide it into segments. This is a general concept, a way of thinking about the race, not necessarily a way you will attack the race come race day (that would be your race strategy). For instance, a 5K race can be divided into three 1-mile segments. Your 10K can be handled as two 3-milers; your half marathon as two 6½-mile runs; and your marathon as two half marathons or two 10-milers and a 10K.

These divisions are better than thinking about the race as a whole. But if you are smart, you will think about your race in segments that cor-

Race-Day Breakfast?

Should you eat breakfast before your morning race?

That depends on the race distance and you. If you are racing a 5K or 10K, food is optional. If your race distance is a half marathon or marathon, you should definitely eat a few hours before race time.

How can you tell if you need food before a 5K or 10K? This is entirely subjective, but one way you can get a handle on things is to monitor your Saturday morning long run during training. Do you wake up hungry and in need of food on those mornings? If so, you might consider a snack—a banana, toast, and jelly—before heading out the door on race morning. Of course, this decision should be made weeks ahead of time, so you can practice eating and running in the morning.

As far as the prerace breakfast for the half marathon and marathon is concerned, this should also be something you have tinkered with during training, so that on race morning you eat confidently, knowing that the calories you consume will be easy on your stomach, and also fuel you to a PR.

respond to the overall effort involved in covering the distance. They are as follows:

5K: The first two miles, then the last mile.

10K: The first four miles, then the last two miles.

HALF MARATHON: The first 10 miles, then the last three miles.

MARATHON: The first 6 miles, then the middle 14 miles, then the last 6 miles.

HAVE A RACE STRATEGY

What should be your race strategy? That depends on the type of training you have done and how you feel coming into race day. If you have followed a training schedule in this book and taken care to rest and recover as race day approached, you should be ready to run these strategies for these races:

5K: Even pace—at PR pace—for 3.1 miles. This is the most efficient use of your energy for a 5K.

10K: Even pace—at PR pace—for 6.2 miles. This is the most efficient use of your energy for a 10K.

HALF MARATHON: Even pace—at PR pace—for 13.1 miles. This is the most efficient use of your energy for a half marathon.

MARATHON: The marathon is different from the other three race distances, since an even-paced race will not work for your PR time goals. That's because every recreational marathoner slows down over the last 6 or 8 miles. It's inevitable. Therefore, for your race strategy, you need to build up a "time cushion" before you hit this point. You do this by averaging a pace faster than a break-even pace. (The marathon training programs in this book have you training at a pace that is 10 seconds per mile faster than even pace for your PR.) Then, when you get to the inevitable slowdown over the last 6 or 8 miles, your strategy should be to hold on, keeping a slower, but still consistent, pace. This will be tough (you are running the miles that make the marathon infamous here). But if you don't panic at your slowing mile splits, and keep in mind that you have built up a substantial time cushion, you should be strong enough to hold on over the final miles and get to the finish line under your PR goal.

BAD PATCHES

Because distance running is hard work and it hurts, at certain points during your race you will be struck with a lack of energy and confidence. These moments are called "bad patches," and they need to be dealt with as soon as possible or they can linger, and cause a massive slowdown in pace. What should you do when you encounter a bad patch? First of all, try to keep running at your designated pace. Then work through some relaxation motions—like shaking your arms out, keeping your thumbs loose, keeping your lower lip loose—while you remind yourself of all the hard work you have done in training and the fact that you are on pace to PR.

If that doesn't work, don't slow down. Instead, speed up. Try a gradual increase in pace for 100 yards or so, then come back to race pace. You should be more comfortable when you get back on race pace, and your bad patch will simply be a bad memory.

THE MIDDLE MILES MALAISE

Different from a bad patch, the "middle miles malaise" is a loss of focus during these crucial miles of your race (most often it strikes just after you have reached the halfway point). If left unchecked, it can slow down your race pace so that a PR is out of the question.

If you feel the middle miles malaise coming on, concentrate on your stride cadence and remind yourself of all the hard work you put into training. Then, when you reach the next mile marker, note your time and make it your only goal to run the next mile on pace. Do the same for the next mile. And the next. Until you have kicked the middle miles malaise out of your system.

FUEL AND FLUIDS

For fluids and fuel, the key is to drink and eat during training so you are comfortable with them in the race. First off, that means figuring out what kinds of fluids and fuel will be available at your race. You can do this by calling ahead and speaking to race organizers, or check the race website. Once you know the type of energy drink, for instance, that will be offered during your race, you can stockpile it at home, and get used to drinking it during your training runs. A good time to do this is during your Saturday morning long runs, the runs that most closely resemble the race at hand.

Fuel can be handled in the same way. Find out what—if any—fuel will be available during your marathon (for example, Gu), stockpile it at home, then get used to it during your Saturday morning long runs.

You also have another option with fuel: You can bring your own—and this might be your only option during a half marathon. If you are particularly comfortable with one type of gel, for instance, you might consider

Make It Fluid at Your Station

The goal at a fluid station is not to see how quickly you can gulp down a cup of Gatorade while running. The goal is to get all needed fluids down, before continuing on your way. Follow these rules to make your fluid stations fluid:

1. Slow down as you enter.

2. Figure out what fluid you want—water or an energy replacement drink—and direct yourself to that table.

3. By waving a hand and making eye contact with a volunteer, indicate which cup you will be taking.

4. Grab your cup and move down the road a few strides, away from the congestion of the water station, before starting to drink.

5. Slow down or stop to drink.

6. Pinch the top of the cup to form a funnel and drink from the side of your mouth.

7. When finished, pitch the cup to the side of the road or into a waste barrel if nearby.

8. If you spill your fluids, go back and try again. You will make up the lost time by being hydrated and fueled when it counts.

taking them along for the run by pinning them to your shorts or the bottom of your singlet.

In general, here are your fluid and fuel priorities depending on race distance:

5K: No need for fluids or fuel.

10K: No need for fluids or fuel. (If it is a warm day, a cup of water halfway can help invigorate you.)

HALF MARATHON: Fluids should be taken. Fuel can be used if you will be out on the course for more than 2 hours. For instance, pop a gel as you approach 10 miles and have only a 5K to go.

MARATHON: Fluids and fuel need to be taken. In general, fluid stations come along every 2 to 3 miles, offering water and an energy replacement drink. Figure out during your long runs which kind of drink you will be taking and when. Similarly, figure out what type of fuel you will be taking and when, making sure to save fuel for the final 6 miles, when you will need it most.

RACE UNIFORM

One way to help motivate yourself on race day is to wear a special race uniform. It should consist of a singlet and shorts, but can also include special socks (a pair that is particularly snug) or a special hat. These items should be rarely used (they have been "resting up" for race day) but, when donned, should help you feel fast, fit, and ready to PR.

The best way to ensure that you have a good race uniform is to purchase a slightly smaller cut of shorts and singlet than you normally train in. (For example, if you run in medium shorts that tend to be baggy, go for medium shorts that aren't baggy.) Then lay those items aside while you train through the Road Work and Strength Work phases of the PR program. When you reach the Track Work phase, wear your "race uniform" for one track workout per week. This will help you break in your race uniform but also make your singlet and shorts something special and something you feel fast in come race day—since you have only worn them during a few track workouts.

Shoes are the final item for your race uniform. First of all, you need to decide if you want a new pair of shoes on your feet come race day. Many runners feel most comfortable with the shoes they have been training in all along. Because they are well broken in, you are certain not to get blisters or feel a little pinching or rubbing sensation at, say, mile nine of your half marathon. But because they are well broken in, they probably don't have the bounce they once had, and you could feel like you are running on cardboard at, say, mile nine of your half marathon.

If you decide to go with new shoes for your race day, pick the same model and size you have been training in, and break them in the same way you did your race uniform—saving them for track workouts during the Track Work phase of your training program. (Runners who are training for a 5K or 10K and consider themselves light on their feet, could substitute lightweight trainers or racing flats here: This will make you feel even faster. However, half marathoners and marathoners should stick with racing in the same model as their training shoes.)

Postrace

Just as you need a race strategy to achieve a PR on race day, you will need a postrace strategy to help you recover after your effort (and maybe prepare you for another race down the line). The duration of your recovery depends on race distance. Use the following as a guide:

5K: Jog 1 to 2 miles after your race, and follow with some light stretching. Have a recovery snack, and follow with a postrace recovery meal within two hours. Take the following day off. Jog easy (with days off) for the next week.

If you want to race for another 5K PR, pick one week from your Track Work phase and repeat the workouts. Then follow a Race Week schedule to prepare you to race again.

This cycle can be repeated three more times before you will need to go back to Road Work.

10K: Jog 1 to 2 miles after your race, and follow with some light stretching. Have a recovery snack, and follow with a postrace recovery meal within two hours. Take the following day off. Jog easy (with days off) for the next week.

If you want to race for another 10K PR, pick two weeks from your Track Work phase and repeat the workouts. Then follow a Race Week schedule to prepare you to race again.

This cycle can be repeated two more times before you will need to go back to Road Work.

HALF MARATHON: Walk half a mile to recover after your race (do not stretch). Have a recovery snack and follow with a postrace recovery meal within two hours. Take the next three days off, taking care to eat well and drink plenty of fluids. Jog easy to finish off the week. Then jog easy the following week.

If you want to race for another half marathon PR, the first thing you need to do is find another half marathon to race. If there is one available, count back from race days and plug in those weeks from your training schedule. For instance, if there is another half marathon in four weeks, count back four weeks in your training schedule (including Race Week), and begin to train again.

This cycle can only be used this one time before you will need to go back to Road Work.

MARATHON: Walk half a mile to recover after your race (do not stretch). Have a recovery snack and follow with a postrace recovery meal within two hours. Take the next week off, taking care to eat well and drink plenty of fluids. If you feel like running after a week off, jog easy for the next three weeks, taking at least three days off per week.

If you want to race for a marathon PR again, take another month of easy, short runs before beginning the full marathon training program in this book.

You need four months to prepare for each marathon, and a full month or more to recover from it. Limit your marathons to two per year.

Well, there you have it: The training plan . . . the racing strategy . . . everything you need to know to go out and get that PR.

Now it is up to you.

Go out there and do it.

Acknowledgments

Thanks to my editor, Meg Leder, and my agent, Farley Chase, for their help with this book. And a special thanks to Mark Will Weber (editor of *The Quotable Runner*), for use of the running quotes in the Training Log section of this book.

Index